W0259341

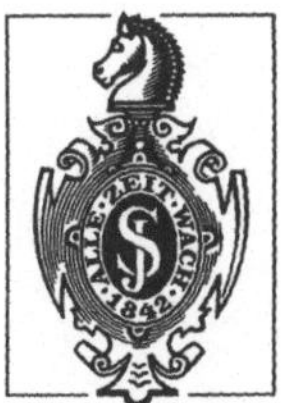
ALLE ZEIT WACH
1842

Treatment of Cerebral Edema

Edited by

A. Hartmann and M. Brock

With 95 Figures and 30 Tables

Springer-Verlag
Berlin Heidelberg New York 1982

Priv.-Doz. Dr. Alexander Hartmann
Neurologische Klinik, Klinikum der Universität Heidelberg,
Ruprecht-Karls-Universität Heidelberg, Vosstraße 2,
D-6900 Heidelberg 1, FRG

Prof. Dr. Mario Brock
Abteilung für Neurochirurgie, Neurochirurgische/
Neurologische Klinik und Poliklinik, Universitätsklinikum
Steglitz, Freie Universität Berlin, Hindenburgdamm 30,
D-1000 Berlin 45, FRG

ISBN-13:978-3-540-11751-3 e-ISBN-13:978-3-642-68707-5
DOI: 10.1007/978-3-642-68707-5

Library of Congress Cataloging in Publication Data. Main entry under Title: Treatment of cerebral edema. Includes bibliographies and index. 1. Cerebral edema–Treatment. I. Hartmann, A. (Alexander) 1943–.
II. Brock, M. (Mario), 1938–. [DNLM: 1. Brain edema–Therapy.
WL 348 T784] RC394.E3T73 1982 616.8 82-10307

2122/3140-543210

Preface

This book contains the papers delivered at the Symposium on "Medical Treatment of Brain Edema" at the Seventh International Congress of Neurological Surgery, held in Munich in 1981. The aim of each speaker was to give a short review of current knowledge in his or her field. In addition, most of the authors presented their own data.

The symposium was divided into two parts. The experimental part focused on pathophysiological and biochemical findings, while the clinical part dealt with therapy for brain edema, with particular emphasis on steroids.

We wish to acknowledge the technical support of Springer-Verlag, Merck Company, Darmstadt and the help of Miss Scholz, Secretary of the Department of Neurology at the University of Heidelberg.

Heidelberg/Berlin

A. Hartmann
M. Brock

Contents

List of Senior Authors

Baethmann, A.: Institut für Chirurgische Forschung, Klinikum Großhadern, Ludwig-Maximilian-Universität München, Marchioninistrasse 15, D-8000 München 70, FRG

Berndt, S. F.: Neurologische Abteilung im Landeshospital, St. Vinzenzkrankenhaus II, Kisau 14, D-4790 Paderborn, FRG

Buttinger, C.: Neurochirurgische Universitätsklinik, Uferstrasse 44, D-6900 Heidelberg, FRG

Faupel, G.: Rehabilitationskrankenhaus Langensteinbach, D-7516 Langensteinbach, FRG

Gobiet, W.: Neurologische Spezialklinik, Haus Niedersachsen, Postfach 280, D-3253 Hessisch-Oldendorf, FRG

Hossmann, K.-A.: Max-Planck-Institut für Hirnforschung, Forschungsstelle für Hirnkreislaufforschung, Ostmerheimer Strasse 200, D-5000 Köln 91, FRG

Klein, H. J.: Neurochirurgische Abteilung der Universität Ulm, Bezirkskrankenhaus Günzburg, Reisenburger Strasse 2, D-8870 Günzburg, FRG

Lanksch, W. R.: Neurochirurgische Klinik, Klinikum Großhadern, Ludwig-Maximilian-Universität München, Marchioninistrasse 15, D-8000 München 70, FRG

Maier-Hauff, K.: Institut für Chirurgische Forschung und Neurochirurgische Abteilung, Klinikum Großhadern, Ludwig-Maximilians-Universität München, Marchioninistrasse 15, D-8000 München 70, FRG

Marmarou, A.: Albert-Einstein-College of Medicine, Yeshiva University, 1300 Morris Park Avenue, The Bronx, NY 10461, USA

Meinig, G.: Neurochirurgische Klinik, Johannes-Gutenberg-Universität Mainz, Langenbeckstrasse 1, D-6500 Mainz, FRG

O'Brien, M. D.: Department of Neurology, Guy's Hospital, London SEI 9 RT, Great Britain

Sefrin, P.: Institut für Anästhesiologie der Universität Würzburg, Joseph-Schneider-Strasse 2, D-8700 Würzburg, FRG

Wallenfang, Th.: Neurochirurgische Klinik, Johannes-Gutenberg-Universität Mainz, Langenbeckstrasse 1, D-6500 Mainz, FRG

Pathophysiology of Vasogenic and Cytotoxic Brain Edema

K.-A. Hossmann

Almost 15 years ago, Klatzo in his classical paper about the neuropathological aspects of brain edema [12], distinguished between two types of edema: a vasogenic and a cytotoxic type. This concept which is still valid and which is the topic of the present discussion, was based on his own and on previous observations. Reichardt [18] already had recognised in 1904 that there were two different conditions of brain volume increase. In the so-called "Hirnschwellung" (brain swelling) the surface of the cut brain was dry, and in "Hirnödem" (brain edema) it was wet. Examples of "brain swelling" were conditions related to anoxia, status epilepticus and catatonia. "Brain edema" occurred in association with brain tumors, brain injury or abscess. The differences in the consistency of the brain surface have been interpreted by Reichardt [18], Zülch [23] and others as a different location of the water uptake. In "brain swelling" it was considered to be located mainly intracellularly, whereas in "brain edema" it remained confined to the extracellular space. Zülch [23], in addition, has drawn attention to the fact that the extracellular fluid of "brain edema" stains with Masson's trichrome stain, indicating high protein content, and that cell elements within edematous fluid may swell, leading to the "secondary brain swelling".

Klatzo [12], on the basis of extensive animal experimental studies, was later able to clarify the differences in the pathomechanism of the two types of edema. "Brain edema" was identified as a vasogenic disturbance, due to a breakdown of the blood-brain barrier to macromolecules. Protein-rich edema fluid leaks from the brain vessels into the extracellular space, particularly in the white matter, the speed of edema spread being dependent on temperature and blood pressure. "Brain swelling" develops in the absence of blood-brain barrier damage; since the water increase is due to disturbance in cell metabolism, it was called the "cytotoxic" type of edema. At the time of Klatzo's description, the most common cytotoxic type of edema used in experimental research was triethyl tin poisoning, but more recently attention has been drawn to the fact that brain swelling associated with ischemic or anoxic conditions is a much more common example of this type of edema [11].

During the past years the investigation of brain edema which initially was mainly based on morphological observations, has become oriented more and more towards biochemical and pathophysiological aspects. In particular, the interrelationship between water and electrolyte changes, the influence of edema on the EEG and on blood flow and brain metabolism has been studied in order to elaborate the basis for a rational therapy of this condition [17, 19]. In the following, a short review of the present knowledge is given, using as a typical example of vasogenic type of edema that related to intracerebral tumor development, and as an example of cyto-

Treatment of Cerebral Edema
Edited by A. Hartmann and M. Brock

toxic type of edema the early brain swelling related to stroke. The reported observations are mainly based on our own experiments, but reference will also be made to recent studies of other laboratories devoted to the same problem. Original data on which this investigation is based, have been published in several articles before [6–9].

Peritumorous Vasogenic Edema

In cats, an intracerebral tumor was produced by xenotransplantation of 4–6 million cells of a rat glioma clone (RG2, courtesy of Prof. Wechsler, Düsseldorf) into the internal capsula of the left hemisphere. Within three weeks, a spherical tumor developed which was surrounded by severe vasogenic brain edema (Fig. 1). Edema was identified by immunohistochemical staining of serum proteins [22], and appeared to be strictly confined to the white matter around the tumor (Fig. 2). It did not penetrate into the grey matter nor did it pass across the corpus callosum into the opposite hemisphere. The blood-brain barrier was leaking in the tumor but it did not break down in the edematous white matter. This could be demonstrated by injecting Evans blue a few minutes before sacrificing the animal. This procedure resulted in deep staining of the tumor but not of the peritumorous edema (Fig. 1).
The distribution of serum proteins, as evidenced by immunohistochemistry, correlated closely with the increase in tissue water content. In the peritumorous white matter it increased from 68 to 82 vol.% within two weeks, leading to a volume increase by more than 70% (Fig. 3). In distant regions this value was reached after three weeks, indicating that edema fluid spread relatively slowly through the extra-

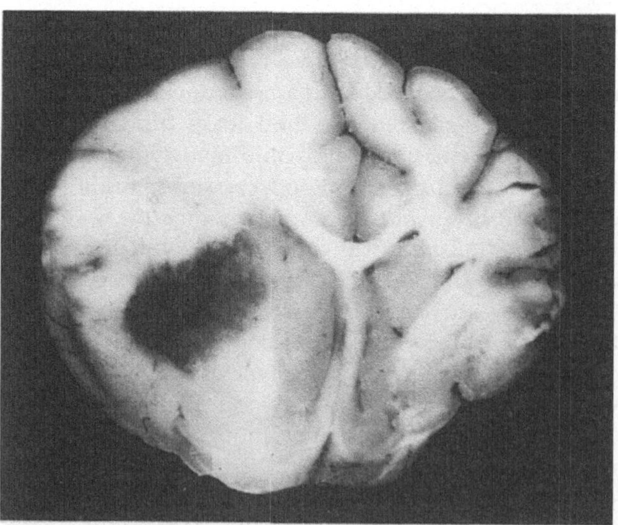

Fig. 1. Unfixed coronal section of a cat brain three weeks after xenotransplantation of a glial cell clone into the internal capsule. The tumor is stained with Evans blue, which was injected intravenously 15 min before. Note breakdown of the blood-brain barrier in the tumor and a massive swelling of peritumoral white matter

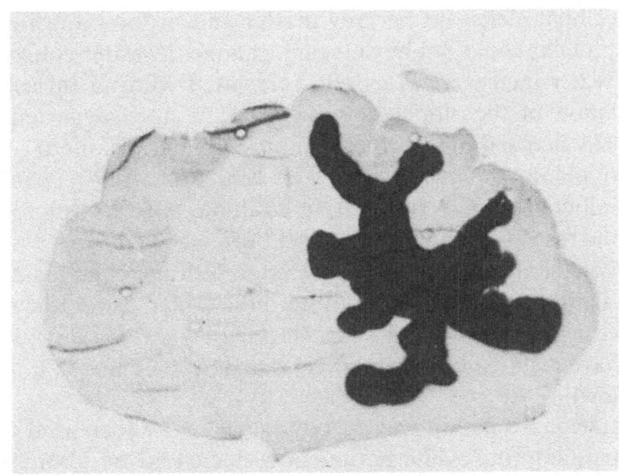

Fig. 2. Immunohistochemical localisation of extravasated serum proteins in the cat brain three weeks after tumor implantation. Serum proteins are visualised autoradiographically by specific antibodies labelled with ^{125}Iodine. Peritumoral edema is strictly confined to the ipsilateral white matter (by courtesy of Dr. Bodsch)

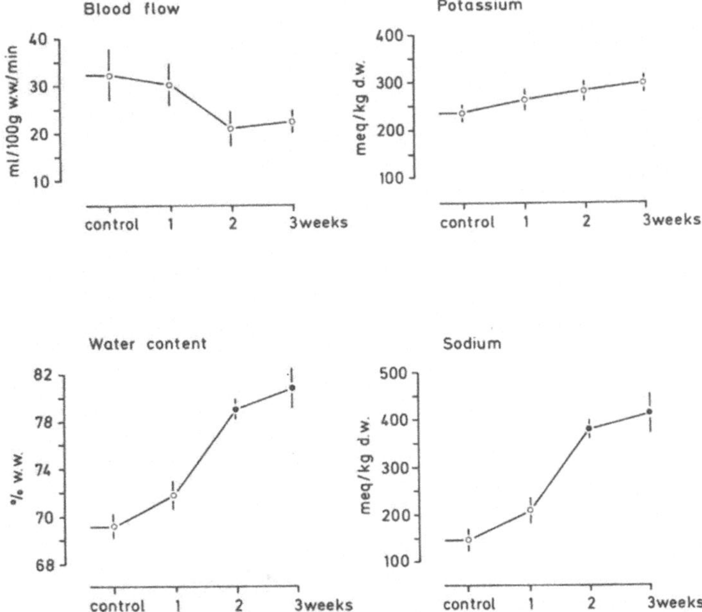

Fig. 3. Changes in blood flow and cerebral content of water, sodium and potassium in the peritumoral white matter at different times after experimental tumor implantaton. Values are means ± S.E. [9]

cellular clefts. In the grey matter and in the opposite hemisphere, in which serum proteins could not be detected, changes in water content were insignificant.
Water increase was closely correlated with an increase in sodium (Fig. 3). Calculation of the slope of the regression line suggested that edema fluid contained 123 meq sodium/l which is approximately 20 meq/l lower than the serum content of blood. The increase in water content, therefore, cannot be attributed solely to the influx of blood serum but, in addition, must be due to a change in tissue osmolality, the reason of which has not yet been clarified.
Potassium content, as compared to sodium, changed much less (Fig. 3). There was a slight increase which is of interest in so far, as it indicates that despite the pronounced hydration of the tissue, cell integrity was preserved because otherwise this would have resulted in a cellular release of potassium, as under anoxic conditions (see below).
Edema formation was accompanied by a substantial decrease in blood flow. In the peritumorous white matter flow decreased by about 40% from 30 to 22 ml/100 g/min within two weeks, i.e. at a time when edema reached its maximum (Fig. 3). In distinct regions of the brain, this value was reached after three weeks, in accordance with the progression of edema (see above).
The decrease in blood flow was not the consequence of an increase in vascular resistance, but it was simply due to the volume expansion of the edematous tissue. When blood flow was referred to dry rather than to wet weight, both flow and vascular resistance remained remarkably stable (Fig. 4). Edema fluid, consequently,

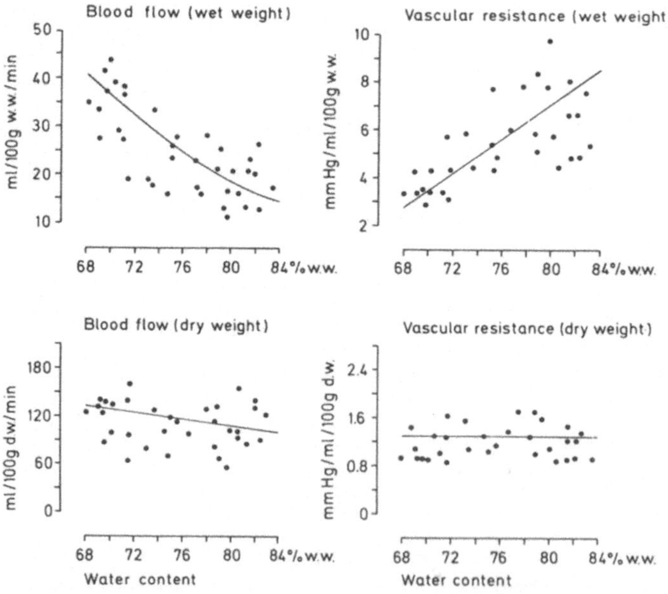

Fig. 4. Correlation between water content, blood flow and vascular resistance in tissue samples from peritumoral white matter. Blood flow and vascular resistance are referred both to wet weight (*above*) and dry weight (*below*) of the edematous white matter. Note the absence of a change in vascular resistance when measurements are referred to tissue dry weight [7]

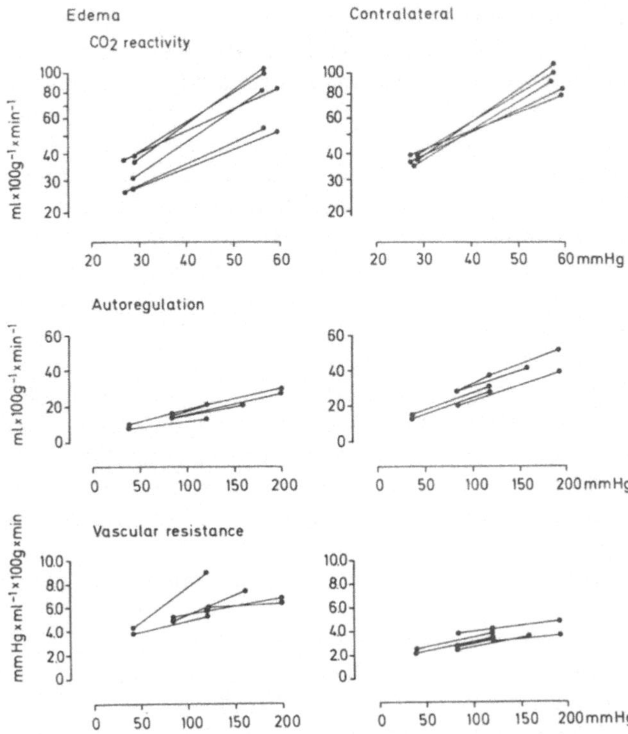

Fig. 5. Regulation of blood flow in the white matter of the cat brains three weeks after tumor implantation. Note the absence of major differences between the edematous (ipsilateral) and non-edematous (contralateral) hemisphere [7]

did not cause microcirculatory compression as has been suggested before [4], at least as long as intracranial pressure was not critically increased. It is therefore not likely that the edematous tissue becomes anoxic, unless the increase of intercapillary distance impedes the oxygen exchange between blood vessels and viable parenchyma.

Regulation of blood flow in the edematous tissue was little affected. Both autoregulation and CO_2 reactivity remained intact even in advanced stages of edema formation [7] (Fig. 5). This is in contrast to earlier observations which have been made in tumor patients, and in which severe disturbances of both autoregulation and CO_2 reactivity have been described, particularly in connection with malignant tumors [2, 3, 15, 16]. In our series of experiments, blood flow was measured using the intracardiac microsphere injection technique, and water content was determined in the same piece of tissue which was used for the assessment of blood flow. A methodological error for the demonstration of preserved flow regulation, therefore, is most unlikely. Unless such an error was present in the clinical studies, it must be concluded that the observed disturbances of flow regulation in patients were due to the toxic effects of the tumor and not to vasogenic edema *per se*.

Edema formation was accompanied in some, but not in all animals, by a distinct slowing of the EEG over the affected hemisphere [6]. EEG frequency analysis revealed that slowing did not correlate with blood flow, water or electrolyte content of the cortex of the tumor-bearing hemisphere. It is therefore unlikely that it was a consequence of compression ischemia due to volume expansion of the tumor mass. Instead, a loose but significant relationship was found with the water content of edematous white matter which suggests that the EEG changes were secondary to disturbances of cortico-subcortical connections rather than to direct interference with cortical parenchyma. An alternative explanation, however, could be retrograde incorporation of serum proteins into neuronal perikarya, leading to changes in neuronal excitability. Such an incorporation was noted by immunohistochemical staining of serum proteins [9]. It was apparently due to uptake of edema proteins by axons passing through the edematous white matter, and subsequent retrograde axonal flow.

Cellular uptake of serum proteins was also observed in tumor cells and in peritumorous astrocytes [9], which corroborates similar observations made previously by several authors before. From a pathophysiological standpoint, cellular reactions to this process may be of greater importance for the clinical sequel than the extracellular accumulation of edema fluid which according to the present study, has little effect on microcirculation, electrolyte homeostasis or regulation of blood flow, at least as long as intracranial pressure is not critically increased.

Cytotoxic (Metabolic) Edema Related to Stroke

Experimental brain infarcts were produced in cats by transorbital permanent occlusion of the middle cerebral artery (MCA) under light barbiturate anesthesia [8]. Vascular occlusion resulted in an immediate flattening of the ipsilateral EEG, accompanied by progressing brain swelling. The latter was continuously monitored by recording the displacement of the cortical surface with a device which previously has been described by Betz et al. [1].

Determination of the water content of the cerebral cortex and white matter of the MCA territory revealed a gradual increase from 80.1 to 82.4 vol.% and from 68.0 to 69.2 vol.% within four hours, respectively (Fig. 6). The increase in water was accompanied by a rise of sodium and a loss of potassium in the ischemic territory. The loss of potassium indicates that the ion exchange pumps were not able to maintain the physiological extracellular/intracellular ion concentration gradients, resulting in severe disturbances of cellular ion homeostasis.

Accumulation of water was mainly intracellular. Cortical impedance, which is a function of the size of the extracellular space, began to increase a few minutes after the onset of vascular occlusion, indicating that there was a fluid shift from the extracellular into the intracellular compartment [20] (Fig. 7). The quantitative evaluation of the extracellular space from the impedance measurements, using the Maxwell equation, revealed a gradual decrease from 19.8 to 12.5 vol.%, i.e. a reduction of extracellular fluid volume by approximately 40%. Edema formation during the first hours of cerebral infarction, was not associated with a substantial change in vascular permeability. The ischemic territory was not stained with Evans blue, and the histochemical tracing of serum proteins did not reveal abnormal passage of serum proteins across the blood-brain barrier during the initial four hours of vascu-

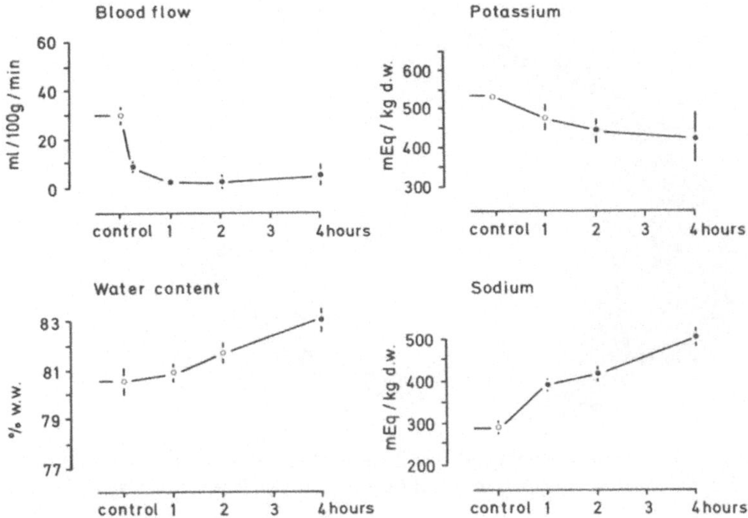

Fig. 6. Changes in blood flow, water, sodium and potassium content of the cerebral cortex in the territory of the left middle cerebral artery at different times after vascular occlusion. Values are means ± S.E. [8]

lar occlusion. Edema, in consequence, was initially of the cytotoxic type, according to the classification of Klatzo [12].

After six hours, however, distinct extravasation of serum proteins could be detected by immunohistochemistry, and after two days massive vasogenic edema was present, covering the whole territory of the middle cerebral artery (Fig. 8). Edema at this time was present in both grey and white matter, which is in contrast to the peritumorous type of vasogenic edema, described before, which was strictly confined to the white matter.

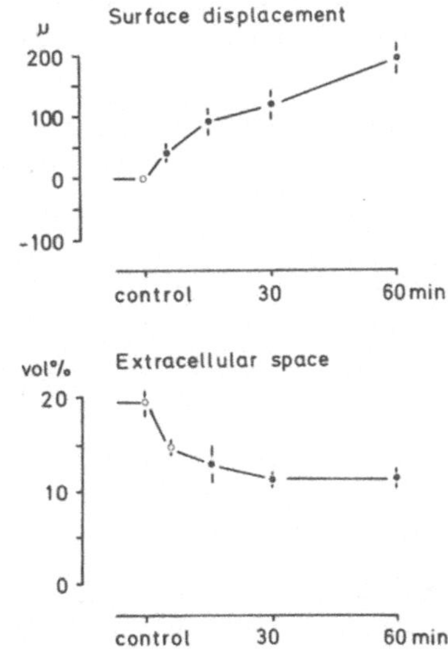

Fig. 7. Changes in brain volume and extracellular space after occlusion of the left middle cerebral artery. Brain volume changes were evaluated by measuring cortical surface displacement. Extracellular space was calculated from cortical impedance. Values are means ± S.E. (closed circles: significantly different from control, $p < 0.05$) [20]

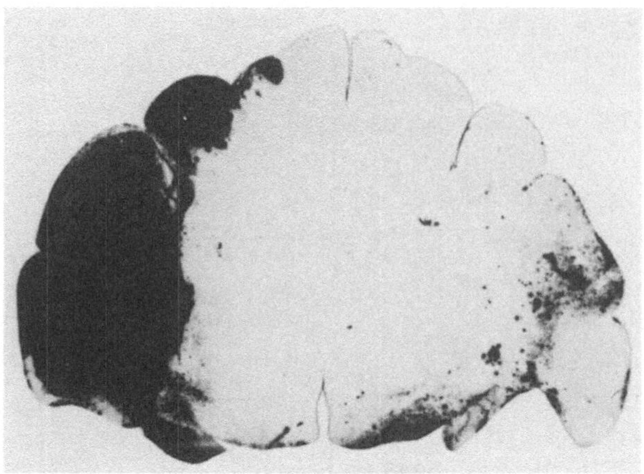

Fig. 8. Immunohistochemical localization of extravased serum proteins 12 hours after middle cerebral artery occlusion.Same technique as in Fig. 2 (by courtesy of Dr. Bodsch)

The delayed development of vasogenic edema after a preceding phase of cytotoxic edema corroborates previous observations made by Ito et al. in the gerbil after unilateral carotid artery occlusion [10]. It is also in line with results by O'Brien et al. [14], who reported a gradual increase in albumin content of the ischemic hemisphere which reached its maximum two days after middle cerebral artery occlusion.

The development of the early cytotoxic type of ischemic brain edema was flow-dependent. When blood flow was correlated with either water or the electrolyte content of the MCA territory, a significant change was observed only at flow rates below 12–15 ml/100 g/min. This threshold was distinctly below the threshold for functional disturbances such as EEG suppression which became evident at flow rates of as high as 30–40 ml/100 g/min [8] (Fig. 9). Symon et al. reported disturbances of evoked potentials at flow rates between 16 and 20 ml/100 g/min, and a release of intracellular potassium into the extracellular space at flow rates below

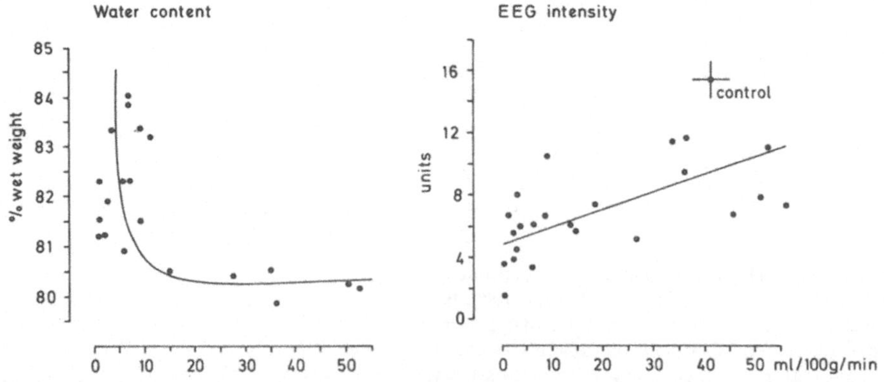

Fig. 9. Relationship between water content, EEG intensity and blood flow of the grey matter two hours after occlusion of the left middle cerebral artery [6]

10 ml/100 g/min [21]. Thus, there is a distinctly higher threshold of ischemia for functional changes than for disturbances of ion homeostasis and brain edema.
The uptake of water during the early development of brain edema apparently was due to two factors: an increase in tissue osmolality, and a decrease in extracellular sodium. Tissue osmolality rose by about 20 mosmol/kg [20], creating an osmotic gradient between blood and brain. The increase in tissue osmolality was mainly due to accumulation of lactate which rose from 1.4 to more than 20 mmol. However, idiogenic undefined osmols may also play a role, as has been described during development of brain edema following complete interruption of cerebral blood flow [5].
Another reason for the increase in water content is a shift of extracellular sodium from the extracellular space into the intracellular compartment. During complete ischemia, extracellular sodium decreases by about 50 meq/l, creating a considerable ionic gradient between blood and brain [5]. During the initial four hours of MCA occlusion, tissue sodium content increased by 30 meq/kg w.w. Since extracellular fluid volume during the same time shrank (see above) most of these ions must be located intracellularly. Sodium is the functionally active cation which counterbalances intracellular osmotic pressure. A shift from the extracellular into the intracellular compartment, therefore, is associated with intracellular uptake of water, which further contributes to the swelling of the brain.
Ischemic brain edema under conditions of permanent vascular occlusion was a limiting factor for the development of infarcts. In animals in which edema developed, flow further decreased, presumably as a consequence of microcirculatory compression by swollen perivascular astrocytic processes [13]. Since during the initial few hours of vascular occlusion, energy metabolism did not break down, it may be speculated that tissue necrosis occurs secondary to the development of ischemic brain edema rather than to the primary ischemic impact, and that vasogenic edema which develops after about six hours, would be a consequence of tissue necrosis induced by the preceding cytotoxic type of edema. If this hypothesis is correct, prevention of infarcts would be possible only by an early treatment of cytotoxic type of edema. Treatment of the delayed vasogenic type of edema then would be useful only for ameliorating secondary side effects such as intracranial hypertension, but would come too late to prevent tissue necrosis.

References

1. Betz E, Roos W, Vamosi B (1972) Interaktionen von Gehirndurchblutung, Liquordruck und Hirnvolumen. Med Welt 23, 579–583
2. Cronqvist St, Agee F (1968) Regional cerebral blood flow in intracranial tumours. Acta Radio (Diagn) 7, 393–404
3. Endo H, Larsen B, Lassen NA (1977) Regional cerebral blood flow alterations remote from the site of intracranial tumors. J Neurosurg 46, 271–281
4. Hadjidimos AA, Reulen HJ, Brock M, Déruaz JP, Brost F, Fischer F, Samii M, Schürmann K (1971) rCBF, tissue water content and tissue lactate in brain tumors. In: Brain and blood flow. Ross Russell RW (ed). Pitman, London, pp 378–385
5. Hossmann K-A (1976) Development and resolution of ischemic brain swelling. In: Dynamics of brain edema. Pappius HM, Feindel W (eds). Springer, Berlin Heidelberg New York, pp 219–227

6. Hossmann K-A (1979) The effect of peritumorous (vasogenic) brain edema on blood flow and the electroencephalogram in cats. In: Cerebral vascular disease 2. Meyer JS, Lechner H, Reivich M (eds). Excerpta Medica, Amsterdam Oxford, pp 337–346
7. Hossmann K-A, Blöink M (1981) Blood flow and regulation of blood flow in experimental peritumoral edema. Stroke 12, 211–217
8. Hossmann K-A, Schuier FJ (1980) Experimental brain infarcts in cats. I. Pathophysiological observations. Stroke 11, 583–592
9. Hossmann K-A, Wechsler W, Wilmes F (1979) Experimental peritumorous edema. Morphological and pathophysiological observations. Acta Neuropathol 45, 195–203
10. Ito U, Go KG, Walker JT Jr., Spatz M, Klatzo I (1976) Experimental cerebral ischemia in mongolian gerbils. 3. Behaviour of the blood-brain barrier. Acta Neuropath 34, 1–6
11. Katzman R, Clasen R, Klatzo I, Meyer JS, Pappius HM, Waltz AG (1977) Report of joint committee for stroke resources. 4. Brain edema in stroke. Stroke 8, 512–540
12. Klatzo I (1967) Presidential Address: Neuropathological aspects of brain edema. J Neuropath exp Neurol 26, 1–14
13. Little JR, Kerr FWL, Sundt TM Jr. (1976) Microcirculatory obstruction in focal cerebral ischemia: An electron-microscopic investigation in monkeys. Stroke 7, 25–30
14. O'Brien MD, Waltz AG, Jordan MM (1974) Ischemic cerebral edema. Distribution of water in brains of cats after occlusion of the middle cerebral artery. Arch Neurol 30, 456–460
15. Oeconomos D, Kosmaoglou B, Prossalentis A (1969) rCBF studies in intracranial tumors. In: Cerebral blood flow, clinical and experimental results. Brock M, Fieschi C, Ingvar DH, Lassen NA, Schürmann K (eds). Springer, Berlin Heidelberg New York, pp 172–175
16. Palvölgyi R (1969) Regional cerebral blood flow in patients with intracranial tumors. J Neurosurg 31, 149–163
17. Pappius HM, Feindel W (1976) Dynamics of Brain Edema. Springer, Berlin Heidelberg New York
18. Reichardt M (1904) Zur Entstehung des Hirndrucks. Dtsch Z Nervenheilk 28, 306
19. Reulen HJ, Schürmann K (1972) Steroids and Brain Edema. Springer, Berlin Heidelberg New York
20. Schuier FJ, Hossmann K-A (1980) Experimental brain infarcts in cats. II. Ischemic brain edema. Stroke 11, 593–601
21. Symon L, Branston NM, Chikovani O (1979) Ischemic brain edema following middle cerebral artery occlusion in baboons: Relationship between regional cerebral water content and blood flow at 1 to 2 hours. Stroke 10, 184–191
22. Wilmes F, Hossmann K-A (1979) A specific immunofluorescence technique for the demonstration of vasogenic brain edema in paraffin embedded material. Acta Neuropathol (Berl) 45, 47–51
23. Zülch KJ (1952) Hirnödem, Hirnschwellung, Hirndruck. Zentralbl Neurochir 12, 174–186

The Brain Response to Infusion Edema: Dynamics of Fluid Resolution *

A. Marmarou, K. Tanaka, and K. Shulman

It is now generally accepted that the release of fluid from damaged cerebral vessels into a space of limited compliance gives rise to the development of local tissue pressure gradients which act to propel the fluid through the brain tissue [12, 13]. The concomitant increase of tissue conductance due to widening of extracellular channels facilitates the spread of edema from the site of the lesion [10]. It is hypothesized that this local increase of tissue pressure is sufficient in magnitude to advance the edema front toward the ventricles where it is cleared by the cerebrospinal fluid (CSF) system, and this sink action of the CSF is thought to play a major role in the resolution process [14]. Our work has shown tissue pressure gradients develop following cold injury, however, they are of relatively small magnitude and dissipate within a few hours [9]. Further studies of tissue biomechanics have shown that with edema tissue resistance to passage of fluid is decreased and that this alteration of hydraulic property accounts for the rapid equilibration of pressure within the brain parenchyma [15]. In our view, the magnitude of pressures developed are more than sufficient to propel fluid through the white matter. However, these hydrostatic gradients can be sustained only with a continued seepage of fluid from the site of injury. Without a continued extravasation of fluid, equilibration of the tissue pressure to the level of the ICP occurs rapidly. For this reason, the role of hydrostatic gradients in the resolution process of edema fluid may be limited.
To explore this further, we utilized the infusion model of edema [11] to introduce fluid of known composition and volume into the brain tissue of adult cats under conditions which did not produce significant increases of local tissue pressure and followed the resolution of fluids containing different molecular weight solids by measuring the time course of water clearance.

Method of Infusion Edema

Adult cats were anaesthetized with pentobarbital (30 mg/kg I.P.) paralyzed with gallamine (20 mg/kg I.V.) intubated and mechanically ventilated on a N_2O gas mixture using a Harvard Respirator. Infusion edema was produced by inserting a 30-gauge needle into the white matter of the left and right hemisphere according to stereotaxic coordinates (19 AP, 9.0 LAT, 21.5 V). The needle was connected to a motorized syringe pump using stiff polyethelene tubing of low compliance. A pres-

* This work was supported by Grant No. 1131624225A2 from the National Institute of Health and the Department of Neurosurgery of the Albert Einstein College of Medicine

Treatment of Cerebral Edema
Edited by A. Hartmann and M. Brock

sure gauge (Statham P23-DE) was positioned in the infusion line for measurement of inflow pressure. The entire infusion system consisting of needle, tubing, gauge chamber and syringe was filled with infusate (serum/Mock CSF) and care was exercised to insure against small bubbles of trapped air. The presence of air in the tubing was detected by occluding the needle tip and infusing fluid into the tubing at the rate of 0.003 ml/min while monitoring inflow pressure on strip chart. With a properly filled system, the rate of pressure rise with occluded needle tip was about 50 mm Hg/10 sec. A rate of pressure rise less than this value indicated a leak or presence of trapped air which, if present, was eliminated by careful re-flushing of the system. By this technique, the inflow pressure during infusion of fluid into brain was an accurate indication of local tissue pressure of the lesion site.

Using this method, a total of 0.25 ml of cat serum was infused in the left hemisphere at an average inflow rate of 0.1 ml/hr. The rate of inflow at the start of the experiment was adjusted to 0.75 μl/min for 30 minutes, 1.5 μl/min for one hour and finally to 3 μl/min for the remainder of the experiment until the total inflow volume of 0.25 ml in each hemisphere was reached. The serum was derived from a blood sample obtained from each animal 30 minutes after initial anaesthesia. Similarly, in the right hemisphere at the symmetrically placed infusion site, we infused 0.25 ml of Mock cerebrospinal fluid at the same rate.

This bilateral infusion method permitted us to compare water content of fluids with different composition at symmetrical tissue sites in an experimental model where rate of edema and total edema fluid volume were known. The time course of cisterna magna pressure (CMP) and blood pressure (BP) were monitored throughout the experimental period. Animals were divided into 4 groups and sacrificed 0, 24, 72 hrs. and 8 days post infusion. Upon sacrifice brains were removed rapidly and sealed in a dry glass container surrounded with finely chipped ice. When the brain was firm, the brain was sectioned and microsurgical instruments used to obtain samples of cortex and white matter of each hemisphere. Tissue samples were rapidly immersed into liquid gradients for determination of specific gravity using techniques described elsewhere [8]. The specific gravity values were converted to units of gm H_2O/gm tissue.

Results

Recordings obtained during the course of the infusion showed that arterial pressure and PCO_2 remained stable throughout the duration of the experiment and no difficulty was experienced in maintaining physiologic stability of the animal.

At the start of infusion under conditions of constant inflow (0.375 μl/min), the tissue pressure monitored by the in-line pressure gauge increased rapidly and peaked at approximately 30 mm Hg. This was followed by a plateau and gradual decrease with eventual stabilization to a level of 7 to 10 mm Hg above CMP level. The tissue pressure waveform during this initial phase was relatively flat with no clear respiratory or cardiac pulsations evident. As time progressed, and with further accumulation of edema within the tissue, the amplitude of the tissue pressure respiratory pulse gradually increased. The magnitude of the respiratory component at an accumulated volume of 0.20 ml was equal in magnitude to the respiratory component of ICP measured in the cisterna magna. The cisterna magna pressure prior to infusion averaged 5.9±0.9 SD mm Hg and gradually increased to a level of 10.3±1.5 SD mm Hg as the total accumulated volume approached 0.5 ml.

Brain Tissue Water

The spatial distribution of tissue water resulting from this model was restricted to the white matter and similar to the profile following cryogenic injury. In fact, the volume and flow rate were purposely selected to match the water distribution following cold injury.

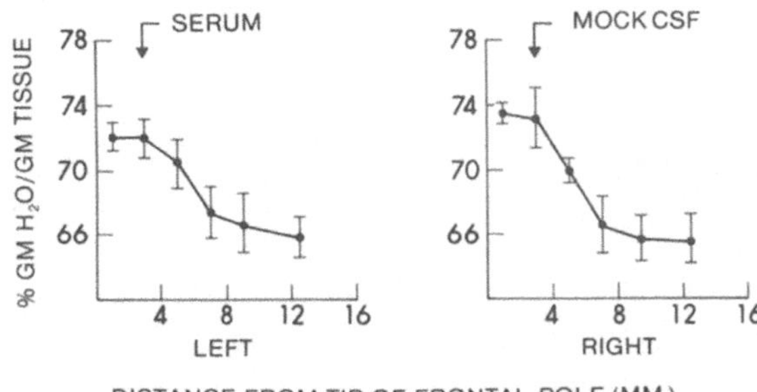

Fig. 1. Brain tissue water content determined by gravimetric methods measured immediately following infusion of 0.25 ml serum (left hemisphere) and 0.25 ml Mock CSF (right hemisphere), distance from tip of frontal pole (M.M))

In animals sacrificed upon completion of the infusion (Group I, $n=3$, 0 Hours Post Infusion) tissue water measured by gravimetric technique was maximum in the vicinity of the infused site in both hemispheres (left serum 72.1±2.17 SD, % gm H_2O/gm tissue, right Mock CSF 73.6±0.66 SD) (Fig. 1). These water levels corresponded to measured specific gravity ($SPGR_t$) of 1.036±.002 SD and 1.034 ±.0005 SD, respectively.

The maximum tissue water ranged from 6 to 8% above normal level at the tip of the frontal pole and gradually decreased to normal level (Left 65.9±2.52 SD, Right 65.5±3.31 SD) at a distance of about 12 mm from the infusion site. The corresponding specific gravity values of normal tissue equaled 1.044±.003 SD and 1.044±.004 SD, respectively. In general, the spatial distribution of water measured in serum and Mock CSF infused hemispheres was similar.

In animals sacrificed at 24 hours (Group II, $n=3$) the maximum water content of the serum infused hemispheres averaged 73.1±0.84% gm H_2O/gm tissue ($SPGR_t$= 1.034±.001 SD) indicating a mild increase of tissue water above the value measured at zero hours post infusion (Fig. 2). The spatial distribution of edema in serum infused hemisphere remained unchanged. In the same group of animals, the water content of the Mock CSF infused hemisphere at the tip of the frontal pole was reduced (71.3±2.2 SD, $SPGR_t$= 1.037±.003) compared to zero hour levels (Group

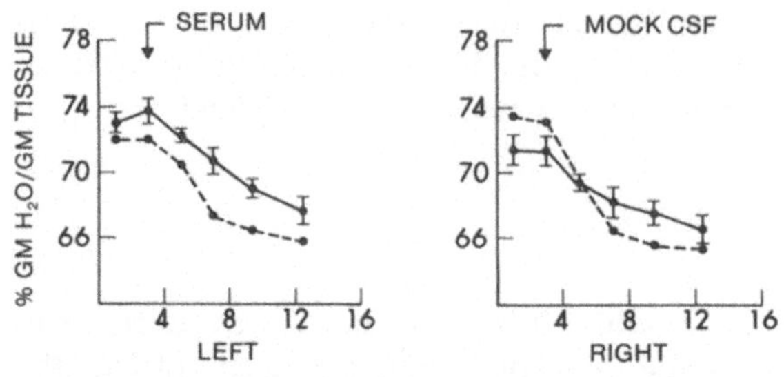

Fig. 2. Brain tissue water content measured 24 hours following infusion of serum (0.25 ml left hemisphere) and Mock CSF (0.25 ml right hemisphere) ($n=3$)

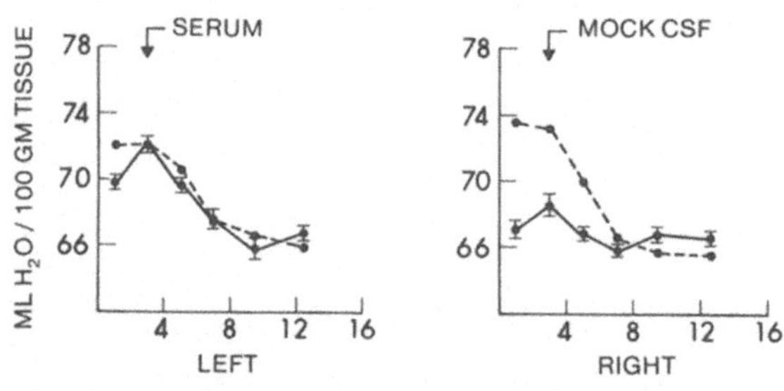

Fig. 3. Brain tissue water content measured 72 hours after infusion of serum (0.25 ml left hemisphere) and Mock CSF (0.25 ml right hemisphere) ($n=3$)

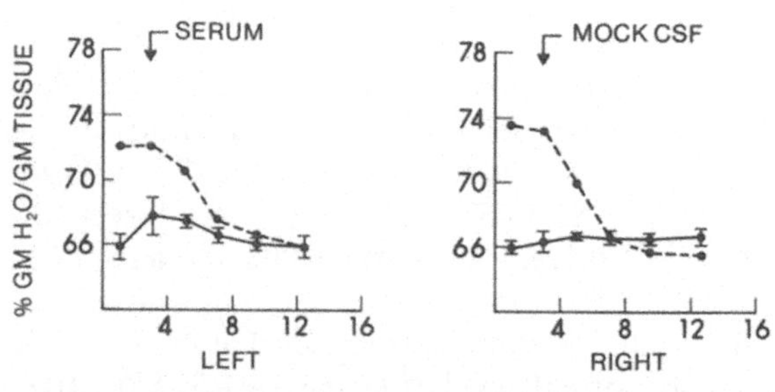

Fig. 4. Brain tissue water content measured 8 days after infusion of serum (0.25 ml left hemisphere) and Mock CSF (0.25 ml right hemisphere) ($n=3$)

I). This reduction was associated with a gradual shift in the distribution of edema away from the infused site.

At 72 hours post infusion (Group III, $n=3$), the tissue water of the Mock CSF infused hemisphere returned to normal level (Fig. 3). The maximum tissue water equaled 68.65 ± 1.8 SD%, $SPGR_t$ 1.041 ± .0021 and was measured at the location of the needle site.

The water content of serum infused brain at 72 hours was mildly reduced compared to 24 hour level. The average reduction of each brain section was approximately 2.5%. However, when compared to water levels measured at 0 hours, the relative absorption of edema fluid in the serum infused hemisphere was negligible. The maximum reduction of tissue water occurred about 2 mm anterior to the infused site (Slice 1) which reduced from 73.1 ± 0.84 SD% ($SPGR_t$ 1.034 ± .001) to 69.78 ± 0.741%, ($SPGR_t$ = 1.039 ± .0006).

The water content of serum infused brain measured at 8 days (Group IV, $n=3$) (Fig. 4) was completely normal throughout the hemisphere. The average tissue water measured in each left brain section equaled 66.63 ± 0.84 SD and was similar to values obtained from the right hemisphere (66.3 ± 0.45 SD).

Discussion

One objective of this study was to compare the rate of clearance of a proteinaceous and non-protein fluid under known pressure conditions. The bilateral infusion of serum and Mock CSF, when infused at equal rates resulted in the development of a transient tissue pressure gradient of 30 mm Hg which gradually decreased to a fixed tissue pressure-CMP gradient of about 10 mm Hg. This gradient of 10 mm Hg was sustained throughout the duration of infusion and was sufficient a driving force to produce a spatial distribution of edema closely matched to the cryogenic injury profile observed in other studies by this laboratory [9]. The gradual decline of the tissue pressure gradient is associated with the increase in hydraulic conductivity of the brain tissue as fluid accumulates. Our biomechanical studies investigating the changes of tissue hydraulic conductance have shown that tissue resistance to migration of fluid decreases rapidly with distention of the ECS [15]. These observations support theoretical studies of Fenstermacher and Patlak who have calculated that the opening of a few (0.01%) channels to 30–70 times normal size results in an increase of hydraulic conductivity of 100–2500 fold [4]. This increase in hydraulic conductivity accounts for the observation in these experiments that a significant amount of fluid could be forced through the interstitium with a relatively low tissue pressure gradient acting as the driving pressure. These findings are consistent with the concept by Poll et al. [16] and Brock et al. [17] that increased tissue pressure could act as a driving force for the spread of edema by bulk flow and the report by Reulen [14] who postulated that a similar bulk flow process was operative in clearing the edema fluid from the brain tissue via the CSF. Moreover, Reulen reasoned that since the ventricular CSF was of a lower pressure than edematous tissue, it was possible that the edema fluid flows down this gradient and enters the ventricles. Work by Bruce supports this concept [3].

Utilizing the cold injury model, Bruce studied the spread of sucrose and 75,000 MWT Dextran and observed from autoradiographs that both molecules appear to move at the same rate suggesting movement by bulk flow. Both Dextran and sucrose were observed in the ventricle and it was concluded that the route of exit of the large molecular at Dextran was by clearance into the CSF.

With a bulk flow process, the rate of movement is independent of the size of the molecule and as a result it would be expected that both serum and Mock CSF would clear at the same rate. The observations in this series of experiments that

Mock CSF was completely resolved at 72 hours with negligible absorption of serum infused brain suggests that a clearance mechanism other than bulk flow was operative. Tissue pressures were observed to equilibrate with local CSF pressure when the infusion of fluid was stopped. As a result, a source of driving pressure was not available in these experiments to sustain movement of fluid by bulk flow. More recent studies by Reulen et al. demonstrated that labeled albumin edema fluid appeared in ventricular CSF when the edema front reached the ventricles and this clearance was dependent upon the pressure gradient between edematous tissue and CSF [14]. It was concluded from this work that entry of the edema fluid is one of the main clearance mechanisms of vasogenic edema.

The results of the present experiments clearly emphasize that clearance of edema by sink action of the CSF is most probably restricted to the early phase of the edematous process when the lesion is active and fluid continues to evolve from the site of injury. The dependence of continued fluid migration upon a source of hydrostatic pressure is provided by the experiments of Aarabi and Long [1]. These workers used the freeze lesion and demonstrated that if the site of cryogenic injury is removed surgically, the spread of edema comes to a halt.

Further evidence that bulk flow clearance is limited to the early stages of the edematous process is provided by recent experiments by this laboratory in which the infusion model was combined with the ventriculo-cisternal perfusion in an attempt to determine the time course of flow of edema fluid into the CSF under known pressure conditions.

Briefly described, labeled cat serum albumin (I^{125}-CSA) was infused directly into white matter of the left hemisphere at a rate of 0.1 ml/hr and at a stereotaxis location used in this study (19 AP 9.0 LAT 21.5 V). When the infusion was underway, a ventriculo-cisternal perfusion was performed for 6 hours using an artificial CSF at a rate of 40 microliters/min. The purification and labeling of the infusate was prepared according to the technique of Hochwald and Wallenstein [5]. The outflow was adjusted to the level of the cisterna magna in order to maintain the tissue-ventricle gradient at 10 mm Hg. The CSF outflow was sampled at 15 minute intervals and levels of I^{125}-CSA determined by a gamma counter. The time course of edema fluid entry into the CSF is shown in Fig. 5.

From the start of infusion and with a sustained tissue pressure – CSF gradient of 10 mm Hg, 2 hours were required for the edema front to reach the ventricular surface and enter the CSF. The rate of edema, adjusted to 0.1 ml/hr, was maintained constant. When the concentration of I^{125}-CSA entering the CSF reached a significant level and the rate of rise well established, the infusion of fluid into the brain tissue was halted (2.8 hours, Fig. 5). It would appear that edema fluid continued to enter the CSF beyond this point, however, when dead space of the outflow tubing and transport delay due to sampling, are taken into account the peak of the curve corresponds to the actual time when the inflow of fluid into brain tissue was terminated.

This experiment demonstrates that edema fluid can enter the ventricular CSF: However, the clearance mechanisms by the CSF route appears operative only in the presence of sustained fluid egress from the site of the lesion. Thus, both the spread and eventual resolution of edema depend heavily upon hydrostatic factors.

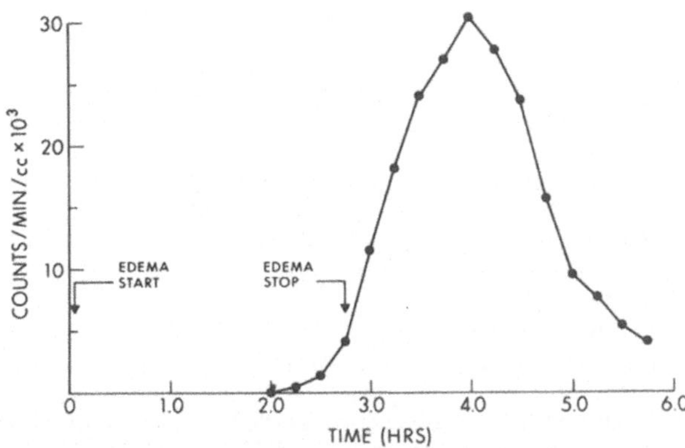

Fig. 5. The time course of iodine labeled cat serum albumin entering the CSF with a sustained tissue pressure gradient of 10 mm Hg. When the concentration of I^{125}-CSA in the ventricle started to rise, the infusion pump was de-energized (EDEMA STOP). When transport delay is considered, the peak of curve corresponds to the actual time when inflow was terminated. Thereafter, count entry into CSF decreased indicating failure of clearance by bulk flow in the absence of a sustained tissue pressure gradient and continued egress of fluid from the site of the lesion

The experiments comparing resolution of serum and Mock CSF infused brain are useful in describing the sequence of events following dissipation of hydrostatic tissue pressures and stoppage of edema formation where clearance must occur by mechanisms other than bulk flow. In studies by Klatzo, extravasated serum proteins following cryogenic injury were observed in subpial, periventricular and perivascular locations suggesting removal of proteins by CSF and blood vessels [7]. However, these routes were deemed of lesser importance than the intracellular digestion by glial cells and it is contended that it is this mechanism which is most effective in removing proteins from the ECS [6]. The time course of water clearance determined by Klatzo et al. following cryogenic injury was similar to the results obtained in the present study using the infusion model [6]. Blasberg explored the movement of substances through brain tissue using ventriculo-cisternal perfusion methods and suggested that serum albumin and/or degradative products are rapidly cleared from the brain extracellular fluid space by an efflux process across the capillaries into the systemic circulation [2]. Moreover, Blasberg's theoretical calculations show that if serum proteins are degraded into peptides and released into ECF a significant osmotic effect could be obtained.

In the infusion model of edema, despite the mechanical distension of the extracellular space, the blood brain barrier remains intact and it is reasonable to assume that vascular permeability was not affected. Under these conditions the increased colloid osmotic pressure generated by the protein may account for the retention of water in serum infused brain. The rapid clearance of a non-proteinaceous fluid such as Mock CSF supports this view.

In summary, these results lend support to the concept that the clearance of edema is initiated by a bulk flow process, however, when tissue pressure gradients subside, we must conclude that the loss of water from the tissue is closely allied to the dynamics of protein clearance.

References

1. Aarabi B, Long DM (1979) Dynamics of cerebral edema. J. Neurosurg 51:779–784
2. Blasberg RG (1976) Clearance of serum albumin from brain extracellular fluid: A possible role in cerebral edema. In: Dynamics of Brain Edema. Pappius HM, Feindel W (eds). Springer, Berlin Heidelberg New York, pp 98–102
3. Bruce DA, Ter Weeme C, Kaiser G (1976) The dynamics of small and large molecules in the extracellular space and CSF following local cold injury of the cortex. In: Dynamics of Brain Edema. Pappius HM, Feindel W (eds). Springer, Berlin Heidelberg New York, pp 43–49
4. Fenstermacher JD, Patlak CS (1976) The movements of water and solutes in the brains of mammals. In: Dynamics of Brain Edema. Pappius HM, Feindel W (eds). Springer, Berlin Heidelberg New York, pp 87–94
5. Hochwald GM, Wallenstein M (1967) Exchange of albumin between blood, cerebrospinal fluid, and brain in the cat. J Physiol 212 (5):1199–1204
6. Klatzo I, Chui E, Fujiwara K, Spatz M (1980) Resolution of vasogenic brain edema. In: Advances in Neurology, vol. 28. Brain Edema, Cervos-Navarro J, Ferszt R (eds). Raven Press, New York, pp 359–373
7. Klatzo I, Miquel J, Otenasek R (1962) Acta Neuropathol 2:144–160
8. Marmarou A, Poll W, Shulman K, Bhagavan H (1978) A simple gravimetric technique for measurement of cerebral edema. J Neurosurg 49:530–537
9. Marmarou A, Shulman K, Shapiro K, Poll W (1976) The time course of brain tissue pressure and local CBF in vasogenic edema. In: Dynamics of Brain Edema. Pappius HM, Feindel W (eds). Springer, Berlin Heidelberg New York, p 113
10. Marmarou A, Takagi H, Shulman K (1980) Biomechanics of brain edema and effects on local cerebral blood flow. In: Advances in Neurology, vol. 28, Brain Edema, Cervos-Navarro J, Ferszt R (eds). Raven Press, New York, pp 345–358
11. Marmarou A, Takagi H, Walstra G (1979) Changes of cerebral hemodynamics in a controlled model of brain edema. Proc. of AANS Annual Meeting, Los Angeles, California
12. Reulen HJ, Graham R, Spatz M (1977) Role of pressure gradients and bulk flow in dynamics of vasogenic brain edema. J Neurosurg 46:24–35
13. Reulen HJ, Kreysch G (1973) Measurement of brain tissue pressure in cold induced cerebral edema. Acta Neurochir (Wien), 29:29–40
14. Reulen HJ, Tsuyumu M, Tack A, Fenske A, Prioleau G (1978) Clearance of edema fluid into CSF: A mechanism for resolution of vasogenic brain edema. J Neurosurg 48:754–764
15. Walstra G, Takagi H, Marmarou A, Shulman K, Shapiro K (1980) The time course of brain tissue conductance and regional tissue compliance in brain edema. In: Intracranial Pressure IV. Springer, Berlin Heidelberg New York
16. Pöll W, Brock M, Winkelmüller W, Markakis E, Dietz H (1977) Brain tissue pressure. In: Intracranial Pressure. Springer, Berlin Heidelberg New York, pp 188–194
17. Brock M, Furuse M, Weber R, Hasuo M, Dietz H (1975) Brain tissue pressure gradients. In: Intracranial Pressure II. Springer, Berlin Heidelberg New York, pp 215–217

Ischemic Cerebral Edema

M. D. O'Brien

The initial response of any organ to ischemia depends on the relative vulnerability of its different structures. In the brain, cellular metabolism is the most sensitive and fails first. The integrity of the blood brain barrier, which is maintained by the endothelial cells of the cerebral blood vessels, is the most resistant and only fails if the ischemia is both deep and prolonged; although the local perfusion pressure is a critical factor, particularly if there is reperfusion of an ischemic area.

The degree of ischemia is not homogeneous throughout an infarct. Furthermore, the development of an infarct is a rapidly evolving situation with different parts of the lesion developing at different rates. All the various mechanisms of brain swelling and edema formation from vascular congestion, through ultra-filtrate edema, to vasogenic and cytotoxic edema, may occur in stroke and the predominant process will vary not only throughout the lesion but also with time [12].

The important factors which determine the formation of ischemic cerebral edema are the rate of development, the duration and the depth of the ischemia, the extent to which the systemic blood pressure is transmitted to the infarct and the timing of reperfusion, if this occurs. In addition there are the secondary effects of the ischemic process on the hydrostatic and osmotic pressures of each fluid compartment and the feedback effect these changes have on the blood flow and intracranial pressure.

If the ischemia is absolute and the blood flow zero, the evidence from experimental animals suggest that electrical activity of the neurones ceases in 10–20 seconds, by 30 seconds the sodium pump fails and there is marked glucose depletion. Intracellular edema, mostly derived from the extracellular space, is evident after a few minutes and by 10 minutes the glucose and glycogen levels are zero and there is a massive rise in lactate. Up to this stage the process is potentially reversible, but thereafter a stepwise sequence of organelle failure occurs as thresholds for survival are reached and passed. The preservation of some circulation would prolong this sequence or arrest it at any stage and, provided that the blood hydrostatic pressure remains low in an infarct, the blood brain barrier remains intact and there is virtually no leak of protein.

Hossman [6] found that after one hour of total ischemia in cats the extracellular space diminished from 18.9 vols% to 8.5 vols%, while the total water content and intracranial pressure remained unchanged. This indicated a shift of water from the extracellular to the intracellular space. There was no increase in the water content of the brain because there was no input. Following reperfusion there was a rapid increase of extracellular fluid and a corresponding rise in the intracranial pressure and water content of the brain; the resulting state being a combination of extracellular and intracellular edema.

Treatment of Cerebral Edema
Edited by A. Hartmann and M. Brock

The timing of any restoration of flow, that is the duration of ischemia before blood vessels in the infarct are exposed to systemic pressure, may be quite critical. Ito et al. [7] have shown that if there is a restoration of flow after less than an hour of ischemia in gerbils, the water content is reduced, whereas if the ischemia is prolonged to three hours there is a massive rise in water content with reperfusion; demonstrating that damage to the blood brain barrier occurs between these times in this model. Branston et al. [1] found that reperfusion after 30 minutes of middle cerebral artery occlusion in monkeys was not associated with any significant increase in water content, whereas reperfusion after 90 minutes occlusion was associated with an increase in water content where the reperfusion had occurred; although this was very patchy and much of the territory was affected by the no re-flow phenomenon. Reperfusion in this way must be a rare occurrence in the natural history of stroke, although it is possible if an embolus impacts and then breaks up and moves off down the circulation. It is of much more relevance in neurosurgical procedures where a major vessel may be clamped for some time.

However, in most strokes there would only be complete ischemia in some areas of a large infarct and some blood flow would persist in most of the affected areas. In parts this would be adequate for normal function and in other parts it would be below the threshold for normal function, but above the blood flow threshold for structural integrity. Symon [17] has reported blood pressures of between 25–40% of normal in the vascular bed distal to a proximal middle cerebral artery occlusion in monkeys and flows down to 25% of normal in this model. Autoradiographic blood flow studies in experimental animals have also shown flows which range from zero to near normal in the territory of an occluded vessel.

Complete cessation of circulation probably occurs for a time after embolisation of a large vessel, such as the middle cerebral artery, but large areas of this vessel's territory would soon be reperfused either because of fragmentation of the embolus or through collateral circulation, or a combination of these two mechanisms. This would apply to most of the territory of a major vessel and could develop in time to prevent irreversible consequences, the outcome depending on the depth of ischemia and its duration.

The brain can survive mild ischemia for some time but it is intolerant of profound ischemia for even short periods so that the depth of ischemia is more important than its duration. The depth of ischemia may be quite critical. Shibata et al. [16] showed no change in electrolyte or water content of the brain following middle cerebral artery occlusion in dogs, but when the ischemic insult was increased by reducing the blood pressure, edema and infarction resulted.

The important areas of an infarct as far as edema formation is concerned is not the area of complete infarction unless this is reperfused; it is the area of relative ischemia where some blood flow persists and in these areas the development of extracellular edema and the opening of the blood brain barrier to macromolecules is critically dependent on the blood hydrostatic pressure at capillary level. With no pressure and no flow, or with very low flows, there is no protein extravasation, partly because the distending pressure is zero and partly because of a squeeze on the extracellular space and capillaries by swollen glia (perivascular hydrops), which increases the resistance to macromolecular extravasation and reduces the spread of extracellular edema. Little [10] has shown that the swelling of astrocytic foot processes in complete ischemia occurs initially near blood vessels and spreads from there, suggesting that the fluid is derived from the vascular compartment.

With some hydrostatic pressure and sufficient ischemia the blood brain barrier opens eventually, but only after an interval of some hours. The duration for which the barrier remains open is variable and also depends on the duration and depth of ischemia and local hydrostatic pressure. Seigel et al. [15] using microemboli in rats showed a big shift of sodium at four hours but the blood brain barrier did not open until 8–16 hours. Klatzo [8] using bilateral carotid occlusion in gerbils found the blood brain barrier open at 24 hours after 30 minutes of occlusion in 50% of animals; whereas if the occlusion was prolonged to 6 hours, the barrier was open at 60 minutes in all the animals. Harrison et al. (1975) using the same gerbil model found that the edema was maximal at 8 hours but the blood brain barrier did not open until 18–24 hours.

O'Brien et al. [13, 14] studied the distribution of water in the brains of cats from 4 hours to 20 days after occlusion of the middle cerebral artery. In this model the water content reached a maximum at 2 days but the greatest extravasation of 99 M-Sodium pertechnitate and 131-iodine labelled albumin did not occur until 3 or 4 days after infarction and remained high for the duration of the study. Comparison of the extravasation of these tracers to water showed continued high levels of tracer extravasation long after the water content had returned to normal. Garcia et al. [3] found peak edema levels at 4 days in rhesus monkeys following middle cerebral artery occlusion with the greatest blood brain barrier breakdown at 7 days. These experiments accord with the clinical experience that edema is maximal between 1 and 3 days after a stroke whereas the Sodium pertechnitate brain scan does not reach the maximum lesion to background ratio for 7–10 days.

The effect of changes in systemic blood pressure may have a profound effect on the formation of cerebral edema though this does depend almost entirely on the extent to which it is transmitted to capillaries. If the major arterial supply to the infarct is occluded, the blood supply to the infarct is from the collateral circulation and in the acute stage, flow will be pressure dependent because the arterioles are maximally dilated by the anoxic-ischemic stimulus. Symon et al. [18] showed that the loss of auto-regulation is proportional to the degree of ischemia, particularly for falls in blood pressure. They found that auto-regulation was partly preserved when the post-occlusion flow was greater than 40% of normal, but absent when the flow was less than 20%. Under these circumstances an increase in pressure causes an increase in flow. Conversely, and perhaps clinically more important, is that a reduction in pressure causes a fall in flow.

If the collateral circulation has to travel a considerable distance, as would occur in bilateral carotid occlusion, there may be auto-regulation against a rise in systemic pressure in responsive vessels too distant from the infarct to be affected by it and this would considerably reduce the perfusion pressure within the ischemic-infarcted area.

If the main arterial supply to an infarct is patent or if the collateral supply is exceptionally good, particularly with small lesions, the situation is rather different and this is because the infarcted area is exposed to systemic pressures so that an increase in blood pressure will tend to open the blood brain barrier early and drive the formation of extracellular edema. This situation is analogous to the cold injury. Klatzo et al. [9] showed that by increasing the blood pressure in cats with cold injury to 200 mm Hg, edema formation reached the levels in 2 hours that would normally take 6 hours to achieve in normotensive animals. Lowering the blood pressure inhibited edema formation. A similar relationship between blood pressure and edema formation occurs in experimental models following removal of/a temporary arterial clip. In these instances a rise in blood pressure usually causes a rise in flow, but false autoregulation may occur. That is a rise in blood pressure that is not accompanied by a rise in flow in a disautoregulated vascular bed. This is due to an increase in edema caused by the rise in pressure which squeezes the capillaries thereby preventing dilatation and the subsequent increase in flow. This phenomenon may occur without a comparable rise in intracranial pressure. Grote and Schubert [4] have shown that cold induced edema can prevent subsequent dilatation by anoxia and Frei et al. [2] have shown that reactive hyperemia is considerably reduced in edematous brain.

Fluctuations in blood pressure may be even more harmful as has been demonstrated by Matakas et al. [11] in monkeys. Extracellular edema was induced by balloon compression, subsequent to release the intracranial pressure rose to a level which depended on systemic blood pressure since the lesion was exposed to the systemic blood pressure from the outset. The blood pressure was then increased with Norepinephrine, the perfusion pressure increased and the cerebral blood flow increased but so did the edema and the intracranial pressure. When the effect of the Norepinephrine wore off, the blood pressure fell but the intracranial pressure fell proportionately less. For example, a blood pressure change of 100–150 and back to 100 was accompanied by an intracranial pressure change of 60–90 and then back only to 80. This effect was repeated with each rise in blood pressure until the intracranial pressure was the same as the systemic pressure and the perfusion pressure reduced to zero. This has an obvious clinical correlation in hypertensive stroke patients with poor blood pressure control.

Although a reduction in blood pressure might retard the formation of edema and this has been shown to occur in the cold injury, in most patients a reduction in pressure would reduce blood flow in disautoregulated vascular beds where the flow is pressure dependent and this could well have a critical effect on cellular metabolism. The optimum perfusion pressure requirements are therefore likely to vary considerably in different parts of an infarct and at different stages in evolution, so that no general advice can be given about the control of blood pressure, except to avoid extremes.

It seems clear, therefore, that the sequence of events in the formation of edema due to cerebral ischemia is as follows. Firstly, there is a shift of water from the extracellular to the intracellular space, which may occur with even slight ischemia. Some extracellular edema may occur, probably associated with increased micropinocytosis if the local perfusion pressure is adequate. Only later does the blood brain barrier open to macromolecules if the ischemia is sufficient to cause cellular disruption and this depends principally on the blood hydrostatic pressure at capillary level. It is not clear why the edema is maximal at 2 days and then improves, not apparently following the subsequent breakdown of the blood brain barrier. It may be that perfusion pressure is inadequate in the infarcted area and that the osmotic effect is insufficient.

References

1. Branston NM, Bell BA, Hunstock A, Symon L (1980) Time and flow as factors in the formation of postischemic edema in primate cortex. Adv Neurol 28:291–298
2. Frei HJ, Wallenfang TH, Poll W, Reulen HJ, Schubert R, Brock M (1973) Regional cerebral blood flow and regional metabolism in cold induced edema. Acta Neurochir (Wien) 29:15–28
3. Garcia JH, Conger KA, Morawetz R, Halsey JH Jr (1980) Postischemic brain edema: quantitation and evolution. Adv Neurol 28:147–169
4. Grote J, Schubert R (1977) The effect of brain edema on cortical oxygen supply during arterial normoxia and arterial hypoxia. Bibl Anat 15, Part 1:335–358
5. Harrison MJ, Arnold J, Sedal L, Ross Russell RW (1975) Ischemic swelling of cerebral hemisphere in the Gerbil. J Neurol Neurosurg & Pschiat 38:1194–1196
6. Hossmann KA (1976) Development and resolution of ischemic brain swelling. In: Dynamics of Brain Edema. Pappis HM, Feindel W (eds). Springer, Berlin Heidelberg New York, pp 219–227
7. Ito U, Ohno K, Nakamura R, Suganuma F, Inaba Y (1979) Brain edema during ischemia and after restoration of blood flow. Stroke 10:542–547
8. Klatzo I (1972) Pathophysiological aspects of brain edema. In: Steroids and Brain Oedema. Reulen HJ, Schurmann K (eds). Springer, Berlin Heidelberg New York, pp 1–8
9. Klatzo I, Wisniewski H, Steinwall D, Streicher E (1967) Dynamics of cold injury edema. In: Brain Edema. Klatzo I, Seitelberger F (eds). Springer, Berlin Heidelberg New York, pp 554–563
10. Little JR (1976) Microvascular alterations and edema in focal cerebral ischemia. In: Dynamics of Brain Edema. Pappius HM, Feindel W (eds). Springer, Berlin Heidelberg New York, pp 236–243
11. Matakas F, Waechter R von, Eibs G (1972) Relation between cerebral perfusion pressure and arterial pressure in brain edema. Lancet 1:684
12. O'Brien MD (1979) Ischaemic cerebral oedema – a review. Stroke 10:623–628
13. O'Brien MD, Jordan MM, Waltz AG (1974b) Ischemic cerebral edema and the blood brain barrier. Arch Neurol 30:461–463
14. O'Brien MD, Waltz AG, Jordan MM (1974a) Ischemic cerebral edema. Arch Neurol 30:456–460
15. Seigel BA, Meidinger R, Elliott AJ, Studer R, Curtis C, Morgan J, Potchen EJ (1972) Experimental cerebral microembolism – multiple tracer assessment of cerebral edema. Arch Neurol 26:73–77
16. Shibata S, Hodge C, Pappius HM (1974) The effect of cerebral ischemia on cerebral water and electrolytes. J Neurosurg 41:146–159
17. Symon L (1967) A comparative study of middle cerebral pressure in dogs and macaques. J Physiol 191:449–465
18. Symon L, Branston NM, Strong AJ (1976) Autoregulation in acute focal ischemia. Stroke 7:547–554

Metabolic Effects of Corticosteroids in Central Nervous Tissue*

A. Baethmann, W. Oettinger, K. Moritake, L. Chaussy, and F. Jesch**

Treatment of cerebral edema employs many methods which, however, do not necessarily influence the processes involved in the formation and spread of this condition. E.g. hypertonic dehydration, injection of saluretics, hyperventilation, or surgical procedures may decrease intracranial pressure whereas brain edema itself remains largely unaffected [6]. So far, specific methods of treatment for brain edema are unknown. Specific methods should influence various edema mechanisms, such as damage of the blood-brain barrier, spread of edema into the parenchyma, secondary swelling of nerve- and glia cells. Moreover, they should enhance edema resolution.

In view of the biological effects of corticosteroids induced in central nervous tissue (Table 1), an interference of these compounds with edema mechanisms is conceivable. Experimental evidence has been provided that corticosteroids limit blood-brain barrier damage secondary to different types of lesion [7, 8, 10, 12] which would directly affect the influx of vasogenic edema into the cerebral parenchyma. Moreover, experimental studies have demonstrated that corticosteroids affect the formation and resorption of cerebrospinal fluid [9, 13], that there are specific bind-

Table 1. Direct effects of steroids on CNS

▲ Blood-brain barrier	Rovit, 1968 Pappius, 1969 Eisenberg, 1970	▲ Electrophysiology	Davenport, 1949 Feldman, 1970
▲ CSF formation	Davson, 1972 Sato, 1973 Pollay, 1975	▲ Sensitivity to barbiturates	Kobayashi, 1976 Baethmann, 1978
▲ Specific binding (Receptors?)	De Vellis, 1965 McEwen, 1969 Anderson, 1976	▲ Tissue metabolism	Hoagland, 1953 Woodbury, 1972 Baethmann, 1977
▲ Induction of enzymes	De Vellis, 1965 Baethmann, 1968 Stastny, 1972		

For references see Baethmann [3]

* Dedicated to Prof. Dr. Dr. h. c. Walter Brendel on the occasion of his 60th birthday

** The technical and secretarial assistance of Ulrike Goerke, Isolde Moll, Angelika Müller, and Sylvia Schneider is gratefully acknowledged

Treatment of Cerebral Edema
Edited by A. Hartmann and M. Brock

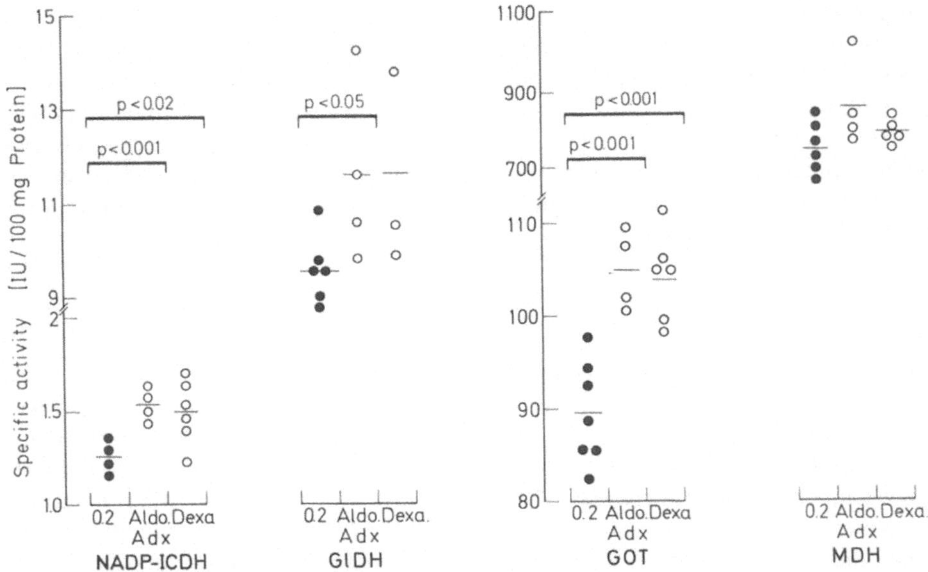

Fig. 1. Specific activity of NADP dependent isocitric dehydrogenase, glutamate dehydrogenase, glutamateoxalacetate transaminase and malic acid dehydrogenase in cerebral cortex of adrenalectomized rats maintained on 0.2% NaCl as drinking fluid without steroids, and after daily steroid substitution with aldosterone (0.1 mg/kg) or dexamethasone (0.4 mg/kg). (From [1])

ing sites in brain tissue considered as receptors, that corticosteroids induce enzymes in cerebral tissue, that they affect electrophysiological activity of the brain, and sensitivity to barbiturates, and finally that they influence metabolic rates [3].

The clinical experience with corticosteroid treatment of brain edema is respectable and the effectiveness of this method has been demonstrated in many forms of the condition. However, there is a lack of understanding on how corticosteroids influence brain edema. This point is not purely of academic interest, but also of clinical significance since better knowledge of steroid mechanisms in brain edema can be expected to enhance our understanding of brain edema itself.

For many years, our laboratory has been involved in research on the effects of corticosteroids on central nervous tissue [1, 2, 4, 5, 14]. Earlier studies have shown that deprivation of corticosteroids by surgical adrenalectomy leads to development of cerebral edema in experimental animals not substituted with corticosteroids. Formation of edema was ascertained by measurements of cerebral water and electrolytes. However, if adrenalectomized animals were substituted with either the mineralocorticosteroid aldosterone, or with dexamethasone, brain edema was prevented [1]. Moreover, studies conducted in parallel revealed that adrenal insufficiency led to a decrease of the specific activity of enzymes involved in cerebral energy metabolism, such as e.g. NADP-dependent isocitric dehydrogenase, or glutamate-oxalacetate transaminase which again was prevented by substitution with either aldosterone or dexamethasone (Fig. 1) [1].

In more recent studies on cerebral metabolic rates, where measurements of cerebral blood flow, glucose- and oxygen-consumption were employed, corticosteroids were found to stimulate cerebral metabolism. In these experiments, cerebral blood flow and metabolism were analyzed in adrenalectomized dogs with and without acute steroid substitution. CBF measurements and determination of glucose- and O_2-consumption were conducted 7–10 days after bilateral adrenalectomy [5]. Development of adrenal insufficiency was confirmed by the characteristic changes of plasma electrolytes. Moreover, adrenalectomized animals had a markedly enhanced sensitivity to barbiturates. It was found, that these animals required only 50% of a normal barbiturate dose for anesthesia.

Methods

Cerebral blood flow was determined in adrenalectomized mongrel dogs (8–12 kg b.w.), under pentobarbital anesthesia three days after steroid substitution was withheld, by extracranial recording of the clearance of ^{133}Xenon injected into the common carotid artery. Contamination by extracerebral tissue was limited by removal of the temporal muscle at the site of measurement. Altogether, four CBF measurements were performed, one as an initial control, another to test CO_2-reactivity of the preparation. Two additional CBF runs followed 30 and 180 min after injection of 0.2 mg/kg of either aldosterone or dexamethasone.

In untreated intact or adrenalectomized controls, measurements were taken at corresponding intervals. The CBF clearance was evaluated both as CBF_{10} (height over area) and as initial slope index (ISI) yielding virtually identical data. Cerebral consumption of glucose, O_2 and of other substrates (β-OH-butyrate and acetoacetate) was determined from measurements of arterio-cerebrovenous (sagittal sinus) concentrations.

Results

A number of systemic changes occurred in adrenalectomized animals which may be noteworthy with respect to the subject of this study. Apart from the inverse changes of the plasma-Na^+- and K^+-concentrations, adrenalectomized animals had a significant fall in plasma- as well as in CSF-osmolality from 307 ± 2.5, or 303 ± 2.7 mosm/l to 283 ± 2.3 or 285 ± 2.7 mosm/l respectively ($p < 0.001$). As in plasma, the Na^+-concentration in cerebrospinal fluid was also found to decrease although less pronounced whereas contrary to plasma, the K^+-concentration in cerebrospinal fluid did not increase, but even significantly decreased [2]. Furthermore, adrenalectomy led to a significant decrease of the blood glucose concentration, although hypoglycemic levels were not attained. The glycolysis metabolite lactic acid was increased in blood from 0.7 in intact controls to 1.2 mM/l after adrenalectomy ($p < 0.025$) while the respective concentration of the ketone body β-OH butyrate decreased, generally suggesting that an intriguing pattern of adaptive processes occurred in the intermediary metabolism, secondary to steroid deprivation. In control animals, glucose levels in blood and cerebrospinal fluid were found independent from each other as concluded from a regression analysis, whereas in adrenalectomized animals both CSF and blood glucose concentrations appeared to correlate very closely ($r = 0.85$; $p < 0.001$).

General Hemodynamics

Adrenalectomy led to a decrease of blood pressure, not, however, below the autoregulatory range of cerebral blood flow (see later). Cardiac output of adrenalectomized animals obtained by thermodilution measurements was found to be reduced by 11% from normal animals (n.s.). However, contrary to normal animals, induction of hypercapnia with normoxia maintained did not raise cardiac output in adrenalectomized animals.
Administration of aldosterone (0.2 mg/kg b.w.) to adrenalectomized animals led to a significant increase of cardiac output ($p < 0.01$) 3 h after injection, whereas 30 min later, cardiac output was unaffected. The delay observed in the response of cardiac output to administration of corticosteroids suggest induction of specific rather than of unspecific mechanisms. Induction of steroid specific effects are known to require a certain latency.

Central Nervous System

a) Brain Water and Electrolytes. Determinations of the cerebral water and electrolyte content in brain sampled at the end of the cerebral blood flow measurements confirmed earlier findings [1]. The water and Na^+-content was significantly increased in cerebral cortex ($p < 0.02$; < 0.001) and marginally increased in the caudate nucleus. No changes were observed in white matter. The acute substitution with aldosterone did not reverse the changes observed, which may be explained by the interval of only 3 h between injection and sacrifice being too short.

b) Cerebral Blood Flow and Metabolism. According to the first measurements conducted in normocapnia, cerebral blood flow (ISI) was reduced in adrenalectomized animals from 38.2 ± 1.5 in intact controls to 29.9 ± 1.9 ml/100 g · min ($p < 0.005$) corresponding to a decrease of 22%. The decrease in blood flow did not result from the fall in systemic blood pressure mentioned above. Injections of angiotensin for examination of the autoregulatory capacity of cerebral blood flow were found to raise blood pressure, but not CBF. Besides, systemic blood pressure did not decrease to a level below 60–70 mm Hg.
Although the CO_2-response of the cerebral circulation was basically maintained, it was found to be markedly attenuated. In normal animals, a regression curve of $CBF = 4.9 + 0.97\ PaCO_2$ (ml/100 g/min) ($r = 0.72$; $p < 0.05$) was found while in adrenalectomized, a regression curve of $CBF = 9.9 + 0.46\ PaCO_2$ (ml/100 g/min ($r = 0.34$; p: n.s.), indicative of loosening of the CO_2-CBF couple.

In spite of the decrease of CBF found at the initial control measurement, cerebral oxygen consumption was unchanged in normocapnia as compared to intact controls (Table 2). Maintenance of normal $CMRO_2$ was afforded by an increase of the cerebral oxygen extraction rate. On the other hand, the cerebral uptake of glucose was significantly reduced (Table 2) for approximately 30% from normal ($p < 0.05$). Since $CMRO_2$ which was simultaneously determined, was normal, the question arises, how the deficit in glucose uptake to fuel cerebral energy metabolism was made up. Therefore, the cerebral uptake of the ketone bodies β-OH butyrate and

Table 2. Cerebral blood flow and metabolism in adrenalectomized dogs. (From: A. Baethmann et al. 1978 [4])

	CBF (ml/100 g min)	$CMRO_2$ (ml/100 g min)	CMR_{GI} (mg/100 g min)
Controls	38.2±1.5 (23)	3.40±0.25 (21)	6.54±0.77 (22)
p	<0.005	n.s.	<0.05
Adx	29.9±1.9 (17)	3.26±0.29 (15)	4.62±0.43 (14)

acetoacetate was studied in addition. Adrenalectomized animals did in fact increase uptake of β-OH butyrate as compared to controls ($p < 0.01$) which, however, was far from compensating the reduction in cerebral uptake of glucose. Hence, for the moment, the question of how glucose was replaced as substrate cannot be answered satisfactorily. The increase in arterial pCO_2 led only to a moderate increase in CBF in adrenalectomized animals when compared with normal animals, while $CMRO_2$, or CMR_{gl} remained unchanged.

Final measurements of CBF and of the cerebral metabolic rates in normocapnia were conducted in intact and adrenalectomized controls without acute steroid substitution after an interval equivalent to that employed in steroid substituted animals between steroid injection and the final measurement. In intact, non-adrenalectomized controls, CBF and $CMRO_2$ remained constant at 35.5±2.0 ml/100 g×minute and 3.30±0.22 ml/100 g×minute respectively, whereas in untreated, adrenalectomized animals CBF and $CMRO_2$ fell to 25.6±1.3 ml/100 g×minute ($p < 0.001$) and 2.19±0.20 ml/100×minute ($p < 0.05$); (Table 3).

Injection of 0.2 mg/kg b.w. aldosterone, or dexamethasone respectively, into the common carotid artery catheter also employed for injection of ^{133}Xenon was found to prevent the decrease in either cerebral blood flow and cerebral O_2-consumption in adrenalectomized dogs. Three h but not 30 min after steroid injection, CBF and

Table 3. Cerebral blood flow and metabolism in adrenalectomized dogs 3 h after aldosterone or dexamethasone injection. (From: A. Baethmann et al. 1978 [4])

	CBF (ml/100 g min)	$CMRO_2$ (ml/100 g min)	CMR_{GI} (ml/100 g min)
Adx + Aldosterone (0.2 mg/kg)	34.0±3.7 (8)	3.11±0.17 (7)	5.16±1.37 (6)
p	<0.05	<0.005	n.s.
Adx only	25.6±1.3 (12)	2.19±0.20 (9)	4.30±0.41 (9)
p	<0.005	<0.01	n.s.
Adx + Dexamethasone (0.2 mg/kg)	34.4±2.0 (7)	3.33±0.32 (6)	4.17±0.56 (6)

$CMRO_2$ were significantly higher as compared to the untreated, adrenalectomized controls studied after an equivalent period. On the other hand, the cerebral glucose consumption of adrenalectomized animals with acute steroid administration was not significantly enhanced, if compared to the untreated adrenalectomized controls. Again, substrates other than glucose must have been utilized instead by the brain. Indeed, the cerebral uptake of β-OH butyrate 3 h after aldosterone was significantly enhanced ($p < 0.01$) when compared to non-treated, adrenalectomized controls, however, not substituting completely for the deficiency in cerebral glucose uptake (Table 3).

Summary and Conclusion

Taken together, adrenalectomy without steroid substitution leads to the development of brain edema, together with reduction of cerebral blood flow, cerebral glucose uptake and eventually of cerebral oxygen consumption. Depression of CBF is independent from the concurrent decrease in blood pressure. The reactivity of CBF to CO_2 is basically maintained, although markedly reduced. Acute substitution with either aldosterone, or dexamethasone 3 h after treatment led to a significant increase in CBF and cerebral O_2-consumption, whereas glucose uptake remained unchanged.

Thus, the experimental evidence provided so far demonstrates again that the brain is a target organ for corticosteroid hormones. For example, the presence of specific-steroid binding sites or receptors in brain tissue, the induction of enzymes by steroids, deevelopment of brain edema secondary to adrenalectomy and its prevention by steroid substitution, inhibition of CSF-formation, and finally attenuation of gross blood-brain barrier damage by steroids, all are indicative that steroids may interfere somehow with brain edema mechanisms. The recent experimental findings on steroid effects on cerebral blood flow and metabolism in adrenalectomized animals as discussed here provide further support.

Based on these findings, steroids can be expected to affect brain edema through a variety of mechanisms.

1. Influx of vasogenic edema may be curtailed by limiting the period of barrier dysfunction.
2. Induction of enzymes and stimulation of blood flow and metabolism may not only enhance clearance of material from the extracellular space, which is contained in the vasogenic edema fluid, but also reverse the primary or secondary cell swelling, i.e. cytotoxic brain edema.
3. Inhibition of CSF-formation may be considered to increase edema resolution by enhancing flow of edema fluid through the extracellular space from the focus to CSF-spaces, according to the concept of Reulen et al. [11].

Obviously, induction of biological steroid effects in brain tissue pertaining to edema have a latency of hours, which in very acute forms of edema renders steroid hormones inefficient during the early phases. However, even then treatment with steroids should commence because in acute forms of edema (e.g. after head injury) edema mechanisms operate which are similar to those forms (e.g. brain tumors) where steroids have been found clearly efficient. Moreover, in many cases edema mechanisms continue to operate, when steroids can be expected to become effective after the biological latency period is over.

References

1. Baethmann A, Van Harreveld A (1972) Physiological and biochemical findings in the central nervous system of adrenalectomized rats and mice. In: Steroids and brain edema. Reulen HJ, Schürmann K (eds). Springer, Berlin Heidelberg New York, pp 195–202
2. Baethmann A, Sohler K, Schmiedek P, Oettinger W, Guggemos L (1975) CSF-electrolytes in two different types of metabolic brain edema. Advances in neurosurgery, vol 3. Springer, Berlin Heidelberg New York, pp 74–80
3. Baethmann A (1978) Treatment of cerebral edema with steroid compounds. In: Aldosterone Antagonists in Clinical Medicine. Addison GM et al. (eds). Excerpta Medica, Amsterdam Oxford, pp 386–392
4. Baethmann A, Öttinger W, Fleischer B, Moritake K, Jesch F (1978) Corticosteroids stimulate cerebral energy metabolism; Support for a metabolic action of steroids on brain edema. In: Advances in neurosurgery, vol 6. Springer, Berlin Heidelberg New York, pp 187–192
5. Baethmann A, Oettinger W, Chaussy L, Jesch F (1979) Corticosteroid effects on cerebral blood flow and metabolism; a potential mechanism in brain edema. Acta Neurol Scandinav 60, Suppl 72:371–372
6. Baethmann A, Maier-Hauff K (1982) Überwachungsmethoden und therapeutische Konzepte beim Schädelhirntrauma. In: Der polytraumatisierte Patient, Peter K et al. (eds). Thieme, Stuttgart, pp 127–148
7. Blomstrand C, Johansson B, Rosengren B (1975) Dexamethasone effect on blood-brain barrier damage caused by acute hypertension in x-irradiated rabbits. Acta Neurol Scandinav 52:331–334
8. Eisenberg HM, Barlow CF, Lorenzo AV (1970) Effect of dexamethasone on altered brain vascular permeability. Arch Neurol 23:18–22
9. Johnston I, Gilday DL, Hendrick EB (1975) Experimental effects of steroids and steroid withdrawal on cerebrospinal fluid absorption. J Neurosurg 42:690–695
10. Pappius HM, McCann WP (1969) Effects of steroids on cerebral edema in cats. Arch Neurol 20:207–216
11. Reulen HJ, Tsuyumu M, Tack A, Fenske AR, Prioleau GR (1978) Clearance of edema fluid into cerebrospinal fluid. J Neurosurg 48:754–764
12. Rovit RL, Hagan R (1968) Steroids and cerebral edema: The effect of glucocorticosteroids on abnormal capillary permeability following cerebral injury in cats. J Neuropath Exp Neurol 27:277–299
13. Sato O, Hara M, Asai T, Tsugane R, Kageyama M (1973) The effect of dexamethasone phosphate on the production rate of cerebrospinal fluid in the spinal subarachnoid space of dogs. J Neurosurg 39:480–484
14. Schmiedek P, Öttinger W, Baethmann A, Enzenbach R, Marguth F (1974) Aldosterone – a new therapeutic principle for the treatment of brain oedema in man. Acta Neurochirg 30:59–68

The Kallikrein-Kinin-System as Mediator in Cerebral Edema, Recent Progress *

K. Maier-Hauff, O. Kempski, A. Unterberg, U. Gross, M. Lange, L. Schürer, and A. Baethmann **

Introduction

Injury to the brain by trauma, ischemia or other causes may lead to formation of focal tissue necrosis and opening of the blood-brain barrier resulting in secondary brain damage, as e.g. vasogenic edema. A variety of chemical mediators, which are liberated or activated in the focus, have been associated with the development of secondary processes. Currently, our laboratory is studying among others the kallikrein-kinin-system (KK-System) [1, 2, 3, 5, 7, 8]. Previous investigations have shown that ventriculo-cisternal perfusion with plasma or with the active principle bradykinin results in brain edema [2, 3, 7, 8]. Now, we report on recently conducted experiments where an activation of the kallikrein-kinin-system was studied in vasogenic edema induced by focal brain trauma.

Material and Methods

Vasogenic brain edema was induced in mongrel cats by cold injury according to Klatzo. For anesthesia, ketamine and xylocaine (10 and 2 mg/kg b.w.) were used. During the experiments, intracranial pressure, arterial blood pressure, electrocardiogram, and EEG were monitored. At time of injury, Evans' blue and ^{131}J-human IgG were intravenously injected as plasma-protein markers and for visualization of damage to the blood-brain barrier. The animals survived the trauma 3, 5 or 7 hours. At termination of the experiment, both hemispheres were exposed for *in situ* fixation with liquid N_2. The kininogen concentration as well as the activity of ^{131}J-IgG were determined in plasma, in focal necrotic brain tissue, in perifocal edematous brain as well as in the contralateral control hemisphere according to the methods of Diniz and Carvalho [4] and Mann et al. [6].

In about 50% of the experimental animals, cerebral ischemia developed secondary to a rise of the intracranial pressure. We did not attempt to influence the increase in intracranial pressure either by using hypertonic solutions or by hyperventilation. The following criteria were used for definition of an ischemic preparation. The cerebral perfusion pressure (MABP–ICP) should be lower than 40 mm Hg for a mini-

* Supported by Deutsche Forschungsgemeinschaft, Ba 452/5
Dedicated to Prof. Dr. med. Dr. h. c. Walter Brendel on the occasion of his 60th birthday
** The excellent technical and secretarial assistance of Ulrike Goerke, Angelika Müller, Sylvia Schneider, Isolde Moll, Mechthild Stein, and Christa Chaudhry is gratefully acknowledged

Treatment of Cerebral Edema
Edited by A. Hartmann and M. Brock

mum period of 30 min or longer, the EEG should be flat and the labile energy-rich metabolites (e.g. phosphocreatine, ATP, lac/pyr-ratio) should display an ischemic pattern.

Results and Discussion

In Table 1, the kininogen-concentrations are given in ng/g f.w. in control tissue in focal and perifocal brain at different times after trauma under normal (i.e. non-ischemic) conditions. In contralateral control tissue, measurable kininogen-concentrations were never detected. However, kininogen-concentrations of 125– 270 ng/g f.w. were found in focal tissue and approximately 400 ng/g in perifocal edematous tissue 5 and 7 hours after trauma (Table 1).

Since normal brain tissue did not contain measurable concentrations of kininogens, it is concluded that the kininogen-concentrations found in focal and perifocal brain tissue, together with the vasogenic edema fluid, entered these areas from the plasma-compartment. The data demonstrate for the first time, that traumatic injury causing a breakdown of the blood-brain barrier provides the basis for an activation of the kallikrein-kinin-system. The question, however, is whether the kinin precursors, the kininogens, which have entered the brain tissue under pathological conditions, were in fact converted to the active principle bradykinin. This question could not be directly investigated because the formation of kinins cannot be assessed directly since these peptides are immediately inactivated upon formation through the effect of kininases, which are also present in brain tissue. Therefore, this problem was approached by determination of the consumption of kininogens which had entered focal and perifocal brain tissue. Consumption of kininogens as a measure of formation of kinins was determined by assessment of the uptake of kininogens from which the concentration of kininogens found at 3, 5 or 7 hours after trauma was subtracted.

The IgG-concentration ratio brain-tissue/plasma served as a measure of the quanti-

Table 1. Kininogen-concentrations ($\bar{x} \pm$ SEM) in traumatic focal brain tissue, perifocal edematous, and contralateral control brain in ng/g FW without cerebral ischemia

Survival after trauma (hours)	Focus	Edema	Control tissue
3	207.2 ±45.6 (4)	171.2 ± 25.2 (3)	n.d.[a]
5	162.9 ±29.2 (5)	389.2 ±117.6 (3)	n.d.[a]
7	124.9 ±21.2 (6) $p<0.005$	388.9 ±57.2 (5)	n.d.[a]

[a] Not detectable. The difference in concentration between focal and perifocal tissue is significant at $p<0.005$ (t-test)

Table 2. Kininogen (K'gen)- and IgG-concentrations ($\bar{x} \pm$ SEM) in focal brain tissue, and perifocal edematous brain in % of the corresponding plasma concentration with and without cerebral ischemia

Survival after trauma (hours)		No ischemia			Ischemia		
		K'gen		^{131}J-IgG	K'gen		^{131}J-IgG
3	Focus	15.7 ± 4.2 (5)		33.2 ±5.5 (4)	7.0 ±1.2 (4)		31.6 ±7.8 (5)
	Edema	16.1 ± 6.5 (4)		32.3 ±2.9 (5)	10.0 ±2.6 (3)	$p<0.005$	33.1 ±3.9 (7)
5	Focus	15.4 ± 2.8 (5)		34.1 ±7.9 (4)	6.8 ±4.5 (3)		40.1 (2)
	Edema	29.6 ±10.9 (3)	n.s.	26.3 ±3.2 (4)	13.3 (2)		37.5 ±9.2 (3)
7	Focus	9.5 ± 1.7 (6)	$p<0.001$	43.2 ±6.0 (6)	8.1 1.9 (5)	$p<0.001$	29.8 ±2.1 (6)
	Edema	29.4[a] ± 4.2 (5)	n.s.	34.5 ±2.6 (7)	13.5[a] ±3.3 (6)	$p<0.005$	33.2 ±3.1 (6)

[a] The difference between both kininogen-concentrations is significant at $p<0.02$ (t-test)

tative uptake of plasma proteins, including that of kininogens into focal and perifocal brain after traumatic injury to the blood-brain barrier. Consumption of kininogens, or activation of the kallikrein-kinin-system, respectively, was analysed by direct comparison of the IgG-brain/plasma concentration ratio with that of the kininogen-brain/plasma concentration ratio. Consumption of kininogens, hence, formation of kinins was concluded to occur, if the tissue/plasma concentration ratio of kininogen was significantly lower than the tissue/plasma concentration ratio of the plasma protein indicator.

In Table 2, the kininogen- and IgG-concentrations of focal brain tissue (non-ischemic preparation) are given as a percentage of the corresponding plasma concentrations. As seen, in focal brain the kininogen concentration was 15.7% of plasma 3 hours after trauma and fell to 9.5% at 7 hours, whereas the respective IgG-concentrations were 33% to 43% of the corresponding plasma concentrations. The level of IgG in focal brain tissue at 3 and 7 hours after focal trauma indicates the level of kininogens which had been present. However, kininogen concentrations of only 15.7 to 9.5% of plasma were found. Therefore, the differences between the IgG- and kininogen-concentration ratios reflect the amount of kininogens which had been consumed, or the amount of kinins which were formed in brain tissue at 3 or 7 hours after trauma. Seven hours after trauma, the difference between the concentration ratios of kininogens and IgG in focal brain tissue is significant at $p < 0.001$ (Table

2). Thus, almost 80% of kininogens, which had entered focal tissue were converted to kinins.

The kininogen- and plasma-protein marker concentration ratios in perifocal brain were almost identical as opposed to focal brain (Table 2). This observation indicates that – contrary to focal, necrotic areas – kininogens which had entered these areas together with the edema fluid were not consumed in perifocal edematous brain, or that kinins had not been formed.

Additional cerebral ischemia secondary to a rise of the intracranial pressure, however, appeared to enhance consumption of kininogens, or formation of kinins in focal and perifocal brain. In ischemic focal brain tissue, the kininogen concentrations were 7–8% of plasma, whereas at 3, 5 and 7 hours after trauma the corresponding IgG-concentrations were approximately 30% of plasma. In perifocal edematous brain without tissue necrosis, the kininogen brain tissue/plasma concentration ratio was under ischemic conditions also significantly lower than the corresponding concentration ratio of the plasma protein marker ($p < 0.005$, Table 2). Approximately 60–70% of kininogens which had entered perifocal edematous areas were consumed.

Summary and Conclusions

The experimental findings presented in this report demonstrate that,

1. vasogenic brain edema secondary to traumatic disruption of the blood-brain barrier supports penetration of plasmakininogens into focal and perifocal brain areas;
2. activation of the kallikrein-kinin-system, i.e. formation of kinins does in fact occur in focal, necrotic brain areas, but not in perifocal edematous brain;
3. additional cerebral ischemia secondary to a rise of intracranial pressure causes activation of the KK-system also in perifocal edematous brain.

Formation of kinins in focal as well as in perifocal brain areas occured in concentrations which may suffice to induce secondary tissue damage involving the cerebral microcirculation and the nerve and glia cells of the parenchyma. Based on earlier observations that exposure of brain tissue to plasma or bradykinin respectively, leads to formation of cerebral edema, the evidence currently obtained in these experiments provides further support for the kallikrein-kinin-system as a pathogenic mediator in traumatic or ischemic brain injury. Methods which interfere specifically with the mechanisms of formation and release of such mediators may substantially improve the clinical outcome of patients suffering from cerebral insults.

References

1. Baethmann A (1978) Pathophysiological and pathochemical aspects of cerebral edema. Neurosurg Rev 1:85–100
2. Baethmann A, Oettinger W, Rothenfußer W, Kempski O, Unterberg A, Geiger R (1980) Brain edema factors: Current state with particular reference to plasma constituents and glutamate. In: Advanc Neurol. Cervos-Navarro J, Ferszt E (eds). 28:171–195, Raven Press, New York

3. Baethmann A, Kempski O, Unterberg A, Maier-Hauff K, Geiger R (1981) Further evidence for glutamate and the kallikrein-kinin-system as brain edema factors. Advances in Neurosurgery, vol 9. Springer, Berlin Heidelberg New York, pp 338–344
4. Diniz CR, Carvalho IF (1963) A micromethod for determination of brady-kininogen under several conditions. In: Structure and Function of Biologically Active Peptides: Bradykinin, Kallikrein and Congeners. Erdös EG (ed). Ann NY Acad Sci 104:77–89
5. Maier-Hauff K, Lange M, Kempski O, Schürer L, Baethmann A (1981) Activation of the kallikrein-kinin-system in vasogenic brain edema; Recent results. 32. Jahrestagg. Dtsch. Ges. Neurochirg., Tübingen
6. Mann K, Geiger R, Werle E (1976) A sensitive kinin liberating assay for kininogenase in rat urine, isolated glomeruli and tubules of rat kidney. In: Kinins, Pharmacodynamics and Biological Roles. Sicuteri F, Back N, Haberland GL (eds). Plenum, New York, pp 65–73
7. Oettinger W, Baethmann A, Rothenfußer W, Geiger R, Mann K (1976) Tissue- and plasma factors in cerebral edema. In: Dynamics of brain edema. Pappius HM, Feindel W (eds). Springer, Berlin Heidelberg New York, pp 161–163
8. Unterberg A (in press) Das Kallikrein-Kinin-System als Mediatorsubstanz des Hirnödems. Dissertation, München

Symptoms of Cerebral Edema

S. F. Berndt

In many not necessarily fatal brain diseases concomitant cerebral edema may cause the death of the patient. Even extracerebral noxae such as hypoxia, substrate deficit due to disturbance of respiration, circulation or metabolism and intoxications may initiate critical cerebral edema (Table 1). The final stage of the most varied cerebral and extracerebral diseases is complicated by edema of the brain, the uniform pathogenetic terminal.

Nowadays according to the mode of origin cerebral edema is characterized as vasogenic edema with damage to the blood-brain barrier and as cytotoxic edema which begins with a impairment of cell metabolism of the astroglia [7].

This subdivision is not possible at the bedside, but it is nevertheless of great importance especially as the change may be very fluid. The clinical symptoms are determined on the one hand by the pathophysiological connections between cerebral blood circulation and intracranial pressure, and on the other hand by anatomical peculiarities such as subdivision of the cranial cavity by duplications of the dura and the consequent constrictive processes [6]. The connection between cerebral circulation and intracranial volume including cerebral edema is based on knowledge already formulated in principle in 1783, the Monro-Kellie doctrine. The cerebrospinal fluid, blood and brain enclosed in the cranial capsule and vertebral skeleton, stand in a reciprocal quantitative relationship to each other in its practically unalterable cavity. The volume of one component can only be altered at the expense of the other compartments (Fig. 1). For this reason an increase in the mass of brain matter must lead to a decrease in cerebral blood volume. The slightest fluctuations of intracranial pressure can, however, be compensated by different protective mechanisms. For instance this occurs through the autoregulation of the cerebral circulation. By this means pressure changes up to 30 Torr can be compensated for by reactive vasodilatation. In addition the extraction of oxygen from the blood is intensified. The increase in the arterio-venous oxygen difference is, however, neutralized by prevention of the diffusion of oxygen in the edematous tissue. The clinical significance of the Cushing reflex – raising of the CSF pressure in animal experiments leads to an increase in arterial blood pressure – is disputed [1].

If the compensation mechanisms described are exhausted the arterial blood supply to the brain is curbed, hypoxidosis develops and the high energy phosphate compounds in the tissues fall away. If the intracranial pressure finally exceeds the perfusion pressure of the blood, a total cessation of the cerebral circulation occurs (Fig. 2).

With regard to the frequency and danger of cerebral edema, it is particularly unfortunate that the doctor in practice and at the bedside has no simple test at his dis-

Treatment of Cerebral Edema
Edited by A. Hartmann and M. Brock

Table 1. The most important causes of cerebral edema

Principal Causes of Brain Edema		
CNS		Space occupying lesion Meningo-encephalitis Stroke Status epilepticus Trauma Intoxication Heat stroke
General causes	Pulmonary	Hypoxia in respiratory insufficiency
	Hemodynamic	Decreased heart minute volume Hypertension Shock
	Metabolic	Diabetes Renal insufficiency Hepatic coma Eclampsia
	Toxic	Infectious diseases Septicemia
	Allergic	Anaphylactic shock

posal for its detection. It is only a few years since localized and generalized cerebral edema could be directly visualized by cranial computer tomography. So far this possibility is still confined to larger centers [4].

The clinical diagnosis of cerebral edema is complicated by several circumstances. The symptoms may be mingled with the symptoms of the primary disease and superimposed by the latter. There is no symptom which is pathognomonic of or specific for cerebral edema. The sequelae of cerebral edema, the increased intracranial pressure can only be continuously recorded after neurosurgical interventions in

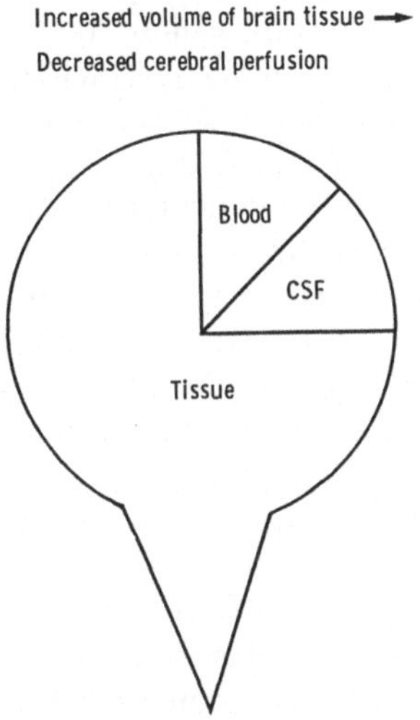

Fig. 1. Monro-Kellie Doctrine: Blood, CSF and brain substance in the cranial capsule are in a reciprocal quantitative relationship with each other. "Guarding" reflexes: Autoregulation of cerebral perfusion, increased oxygen uptake, Cushing-reflex

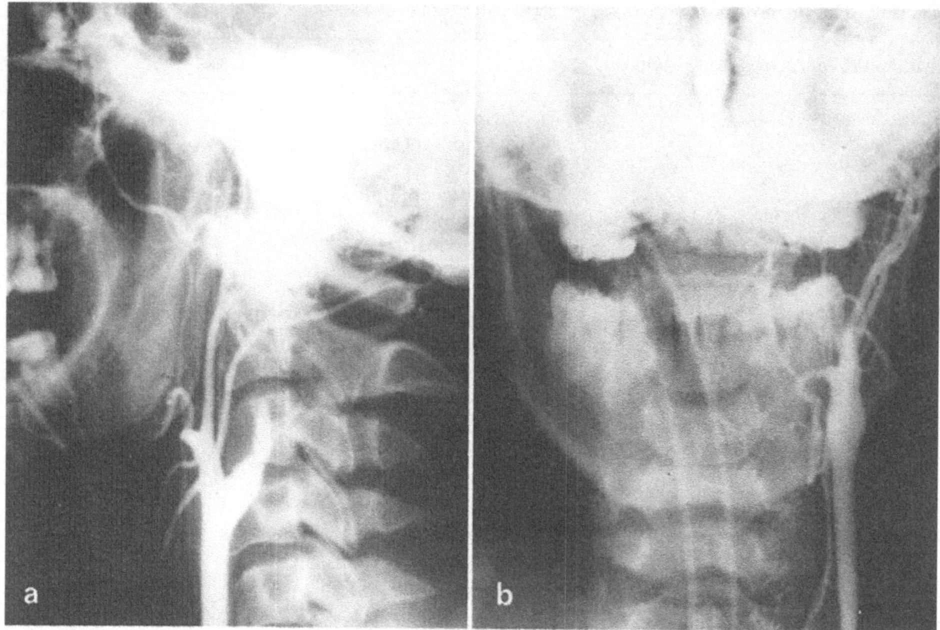

Fig. 2. Cerebral circulatory arrest in peracute cerebral edema. In the lateral and antero-posterior exposures the angiogram of the left carotid shows a rupture of the contrast medium column and a defective filling of the cerebral vessels: The patient is cerebrally dead

larger centers and intensive care wards. Its practicability would be considerably promoted by the miniaturization of the measuring methods [2, 5].

With normal flexibility of the brain tissue and vascular system to pressure and open communication with the CSF system, the increases in intracranial volume associated with cerebral edema are first compensated by displacing CSF from the cranial cavity into the spinal space and local displacement of cerebral blood volume in the region of the venous low pressure system. The CSF pressure remains normal at first. Only when these capacities are used up the entire intracranial space approaches the conditions of a hydraulic system, i.e. the smallest increases in volume lead to considerable rises in pressure.

A lumbar puncture to investigate the nature and pressure of the CSF is contra-indicated when cerebral edema is suspected, since it may cause an acute life-threatening situation with herniation. If no mass displacement occurs, echo-encephalography is useless. The EEG shows unspecific general changes with or without focal findings. For these reasons it seems not superfluous to present in summary the easily detectable clinical symptoms of increase in intracranial pressure due to cerebral edema.

Perifocal edema accompanying tumors, metastases, abscess, or cerebral infarction intensify existing focal symptoms before it can lead, together with the primary disease, to a rise in intracranial pressure. As we know from computer tomographic studies, metastases, abscesses and meningiomata are frequently accompanied by a particularly pronounced edema and are partly responsible for the local symptoms.

The "concomitant edema" arises either on histotoxic grounds due to the metabolic products of a tumor, or hemodynamically by compression of the neighboring veins. Often both mechanisms may participate simultaneously in the production of the edema [10].

Primary space-occupying lesions and edema may, particularly if the process occurs in the vicinity of the ventricular system, cause obstruction to the outflow of the CSF. As a result of continued CSF production the rostral CSF spaces enlarge and lead to an obstructive internal hydrocephalus.

If *generalized cerebral edema* develops because of a diffuse aggressive cerebral or extracerebral toxin the increase in intracranial pressure may also arise without a circumscribed space-occupying process. Here again inflammatory brain diseases, venous sinus thromboses, metabolic comata, insolation and recent cerebral injury may be referred to. With the rise in intracranial pressure a circulatory obstruction develops simultaneously. The venous pressure rises and the arteriovenous pressure difference falls. This results in a general slowing of the circulation which might be detected arteriographically. This retardation of the cerebral circulation leads to a reduced oxygen supply, finally to oxygen deficit and hypoxidosis of the cerebral tissue with impairment of brain function. The cerebral hypoxidosis itself causes cerebral edema in a vicious circle which may lead to arrest of the cerebral circulation and cerebral death.

In generalized edema, the cerebral cortical edema leads to clouding of the consciousness, later to coma with convulsions.

Headaches which are particularly caused by fluctuations in intracranial pressure frequently occur acutely in patients with cerebral edema with or without vomiting. They are among the most common symptoms and are also frequently the first complaint. The headaches are intensely oppressive in character or are perceived as a diffuse pressure.

In some patients the pain is localized frontally or behind the eyes, in others again in the temples or in the occiput and neck. Typically they begin in the early morning and increase when the head is moved. Slight movements of the head may also trigger surges of vomiting independently of food intake. Frequently the vomiting is not preceded by any appreciable nausea.

Besides headaches, *psychological changes* may be a sign of general circulatory disorders. The organic psychosyndrome occurring here is characterized by loss of interest, indifference, lack of spontaneity and affective peculiarities. In addition there are for thrightness, euphoria and disinhibition. Later on there may be also impairment of memory, orientation and ability to concentrate before disturbances of consciousness appear. There is a significant correlation between the severity of disturbance of consciousness and cerebral blood flow as Frowein et al. [3] have shown by serial angiography.

The appearence of *choked disk* is of particular interest as the best known symptom of intracranial pressure. It may be the initial symptom, develop only later or be missing altogether, especially in older patients. It is common but by no means always detectable, when a patient goes to the doctor on account of headache and vomiting. However, if visual disturbances, e.g. blurred vision, increasing visual failure or attacks of amblyopia cause the patient to consult the ophthalmologist, then there is often a moderate to advanced choked disk. Choked disk associated with intracranial pressure is often bilateral. It is enlarged and has indistinct margins. The prominence is measurable with the ophthalmoscope. The veins are thickened, there are possibly striate hemorrhages in the papilla or in the immediate surroundings. The blind spot is enlarged, in contrast to the papillary swelling in malignant hypertension. On examination of 151 patients, Richard [8] found, as was to be expected, a positive, even if not very close correlation between papillary prominence and the level of the ventricular CSF pressure. A choked disk as a rule justifies the assumption of a pathologically raised CSF pressure. On the other hand, in the absence of a choked disk or the presence of papillary atrophy it must not be concluded that normal pressure conditions exist. If a raised intracranial pressure is suspected on clinical grounds, the absence of a choked disk cannot be the sole criterion for the safety of a lumbar puncture to remove CSF.

Disorders of the field of vision are less often found, e.g., a bitemporal hemianopia in the event of pressure of the distended third ventricle or the gyri recti on the optic chiasma. Strangulation of the posterior cerebral artery at the tentorial incisure can give rise to an homonymous hemianopia.

Among the symptoms of generalized cerebral edema autonomic disorders of heart rate, blood pressure, respiration and temperature regulation also occur. The acute intracranial rise in pressure syndrome described by Cushing [1] consisting of the triad bradycardia, hypertension and fall in heart rate, is observed less often in clinical routine than a rise in pulse rate with asystematic changes of mean arterial pressure and body temperature. The reaction pointed out by Cushing must therefore be considered as a special case of the normal distribution of possible autonomic reactions.

The subdivision of the cranium into 3 separate chambers by the falx and tentorium can have a fateful result in cerebral edema (Fig. 3). If the intracranial pressure rises, portions of the brain become wedged in the tentorial incisura and in the foramen magnum due to mass displacement. When the supratentorial pressure rises the midbrain is compressed by the medial portions of the temporal lobes. The consequences of this are coma with mydriasis, temperature disturbances and "extension spasms". Compression of the medulla oblongata by the cerebellar tonsils causes reflex stiff-

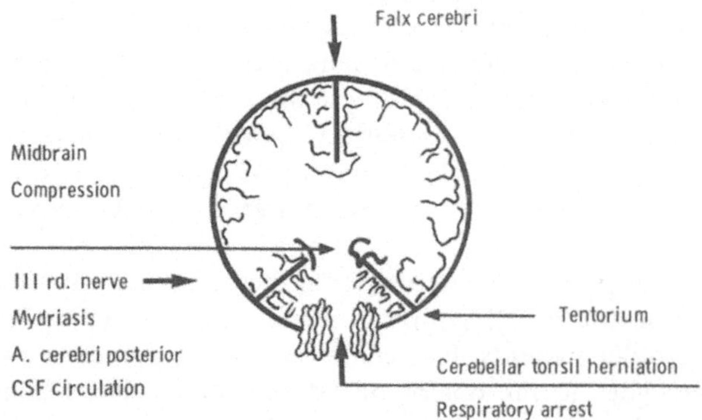

Fig. 3. Division of the intracranial space and the mechanism of tonsillar herniation by intracranial pressure

ness of the neck with vomiting, bradycardia and finally central respiratory paralysis. These dramatic symptoms of tonsillar herniation are often preceded by discrete warning signs.

Compression of the midbrain may be preceded by paresthesias in the trigeminal region. Unilateral *disturbance of the pupil*, usually in form of dilatation of the pupils which may be preceded for a short time by a spastic miosis, is part of the midbrain symptoms. The third cranial nerve, running in the basal cistern, is stretched by the transverse displacement of the brain stem or compressed by herniation of the temporal lobe. As the pupils are further dilated, the light reaction usually disappears.

As unconsciousness deepens, further signs of midbrain damage appear in the form of "extension spasms" of the extremities which arise either spontaneously or on slight stimulation. This consists of a typical extension position of the trunk, lower and upper extremities. The hip and knee joints are rigidly extended, the tips of the toes point downwards, the arms are rotated inwards and extended. This is not an epileptic manifestation but the expression of decerebrate rigidity and consequently a very unfavorable prognostic sign. A similar syndrome can be produced in experimental animals by a transverse lesion in the region of the quadrigeminal plate. Richard [8] discovered that there was a chance of survival only in those craniocerebral injuries with stretch reflexes where the mean ventricular CSF pressure did not exceed 30 mm Hg.

As preliminary and warning signs of tonsillar herniation into the foramen magnum pains in the shoulder and neck region may appear which arise from stimulation of spinal roots of the 11th cranial nerve as the cerebellar tonsils are pushed downwards.

At the same time the medulla oblongata is compressed. Symptoms of the long sensory tracts such as "rippling" paresthesias may also occur in the arms and legs. The threatening respiratory paralysis is preceded by increased yawning. Coma, loss of tone, respiratory paralysis, and circulatory disturbances and the bilateral mydriasis form the picture of the "*bulbocerebral syndrome*".

In their advanced stages midbrain and "bulbocerebral syndromes" cannot always be differentiated from each other. The automatic disturbances are common to both.

In a final evaluation of the individual symptoms with regard to their utility and conclusiveness for diagnosis at the bedside, the symptoms of acute rise in intracranial pressure can be differentiated from the symptoms of acute displacement of cerebral masses. Relatively reliable symptoms of generalized cerebral edema are headaches, choked discs and psychological peculiarities and clouding of consciousness. On the other hand unconsciousness, disorders of respiration and circulation and pupillary disturbances correlate more with the process of transverse and axial displacement of cerebral mass and alteration of structures in the brain stem and the midbrain.

References

1. Cushing H (1902) Physiologische und anatomische Beobachtungen über den Einfluß von Hirnkompression auf den intrakraniellen Kreislauf und über einige hiermit verwandte Erscheinungen. Mitt Grenzgeb Med Chir 9, 733–808
2. Dietrich K, Gaab M, Knoblich OE, Schupp J, Ott B (1977) A new miniaturized system for monitoring the epidural pressure in children and adults. Neuropädiatrie 8, 21–28

3. Frowein RA, Wieck HH, Friedmann G, Kinzel W (1964) Serienangiographische Untersuchung der Hirndurchblutung bei körperlich begründbaren Psychosen infolge intrakranieller Drucksteigerung. Acta Neurochir (Wien) 12, 498–520
4. Fuhrmeister U, Berndt SF (1976) Pathophysiologie, Klinik und Therapie des Hirnödems. Dtsch Ärzteblatt 73, 1601–1607
5. Gaab MR, Knoblich OE, Dietrich K (1980) Intrakranielle Drucküberwachung mit miniaturisierten Methoden. In: Cerebrospinalflüssigkeit – CSF. Dommasch D, Mertens HG (eds). Thieme, Stuttgart New York, pp 238–242
6. Gänshirt H (1957) Die Sauerstoffversorgung des Gehirns und ihre Störungen bei Liquordrucksteigerungen und Hirnödem. Springer, Berlin Göttingen Heidelberg
7. Klatzo J (1972) Pathophysiological aspects of brain edema. In: Steroids and brain edema. Reulen HJ, Schürmann K (eds). Springer, Berlin Heidelberg New York, pp 1–8
8. Richard KE (1980) Intrakranielle Drucksteigerung, ihre Pathogenese, Klinik und Behandlung. Nervenarzt 51, 392–405
9. Schaltenbrand G (1969) Allgemeine Neurologie, Thieme, Stuttgart
10. Scheid W (1980) Lehrbuch der Neurologie. 4. Aufl., Thieme, Stuttgart New York

The Diagnosis of Brain Edema by Computed Tomography

W. R. Lanksch

Axial computed tomography is an X-ray technique which for the first time enables minimal differences in the X-ray absorption of intracranial soft tissue to be measured exactly and their spatial distribution to be represented as a scan [1, 5, 20, 29, 59, 62]. When this method of examination was introduced, it appeared to be possible to detect brain edema *in vivo*. Computed tomographic phantom measurements have shown that water and fat have lower absorption values than cerebral tissue and are in the zero or negative region of the Hounsfield scale. Because of their absorption properties, water and fat have been regarded as the factors which chiefly influence reductions in density in a computed tomogram. Zones of reduced absorption of radiation in the area surrounding cerebral tumors, metastases, abscesses and hemorrhages have therefore been interpreted as zones of perifocal edema [1, 5, 16, 33, 53, 61]. Biochemical and computed tomographical examinations of perifocal edema in patients with cerebral tumors confirmed this hypothesis [40, 41, 42]. Before removal of a cerebral tumor in our patients, tissue samples were taken from the edema zone close to the tumor and their water and lipid contents were investigated. These laboratory data were compared directly with the corresponding absorption values in the computed tomogram. It was found that the rise in water content in the cerebral parenchyma leads to a significant decrease in the density values in the computed tomogram. Comparable results were obtained by Torack et al. [79, 80] who carried out their investigations on autopsy material (see Table 1). It was possible to

Table 1. Correlation of water content and X-ray absorption values in the computed tomogram in perifocal brain edema

	Water content ml/100 g	Hounsfield unit	
Normal value	70.53 ±1.40	18.2 ±1.5	Torack and co-workers
Brain edema	79.70 ±4.77	12.6 ±2.9	
Difference	9.17	5.6	
Normal value	69.10	15.50 ±0.99	Our investigations
Brain edema	78.78 ±1.21	12.10 ±0.59	
Difference	9.68	3.40	

Treatment of Cerebral Edema
Edited by A. Hartmann and M. Brock

Table 2. Comparison of the water content of the grey and white matter and of the total lipid content with the absorption values in the CT in brain edema

	Water content grey matter ml/100 g ww.	Water content white matter ml/100 g ww.	Total lipid content g/100 g ww.	Hounsfield unit
Normal value	81.70 ±1.00	69.1	19.0	30.96
Brain edema	83.77 ±0.97	81.36 ±1.49	13.98 ±1.43	21.48 ±1.7

confirm and improve these results by a second series of investigations with a third generation CT apparatus (EMI CT 1010).

The rise in tissue water content to 12.26% above the normal value (from 69.1% to 81.36%) corresponds to an average drop in tissue density of 9.48 Hounsfield units (from 30.96 HU to 21.48 HU) (Table 2). This relationship shows that the water content in the white matter only has to rise by an average of 1.26% for the corresponding numerically expressed absorption values to be reduced by 1 Hounsfield unit. In the first series of investigations, this threshold value was higher; the water content of the white matter had to increase by 2.84% in order to effect a change in the absorption values of 1 Hounsfield unit. In our opinion, comparison of the results (Table 3) leads to the tentative conclusion that a 100% increase in the sensitivity of edema detection in the white matter of the cerebral hemispheres has been achieved with the third generation of computed tomographs.

These comparative analyses, carried out for the first time *in vivo*, of tissue water content in peritumoral brain edema and of the corresponding tissue specific gravities measured by computed tomography have shown that the increase in water content in the white matter of cerebral tissue correlates directly with the decrease in X-ray absorption values and thus with the tissue specific gravity. These investigations give for the first time the threshold value for the minimum change in tissue water content which must be exceeded for the corresponding absorption values in the computed tomogram to be changed by one unit. This threshold value defines on the one hand the sensitivity and on the other hand the functional limit of this method of investigation for the detection of perifocal edema in cerebral tumors. The question of whether there are cerebral tumors which are surrounded by edema in which the in-

Table 3. Sensitivity of CT systems in the detection of perifocal brain edema

	Increase in the H_2O content (mean) white matter (%)	Decrease in the Hounsfield units (HU) white matter	Increase in H_2O content to alter the absorption by 1 HU (%)
CT EMI Mark 1	9.68	3.4	2.84
CT EMI 1010	12.26	9.48	1.29

crease in water content is on average less than 1.3% cannot yet be answered on the basis of our investigations. Only in three patients with inoperable cerebral tumors where no brain edema was shown in the computed tomogram have we been able to confirm, by autopsy, that no edema was to be found in the adjacent cerebral white matter, either macroscopically or by optical microscopy. Of course the above question cannot be answered by these three isolated observations.

The high density-resolution power of the CT instruments of the third generation and especially of the fourth generation as a rule enables a clear visual differentiation between grey and white matter in the analogue image under optimum investigation conditions (absolutely artefact-free analogue images). In the digital print-out, different absorption values result from the correspondingly different shades of grey for the white and grey matter in the analogue image.

There is a difference of about 6 Hounsfield units between the mean absorption values of grey and white matter. This difference corresponds to the Hounsfield units for grey and white matter given by Arimitsu et al. [2]. The lower absorption values for white matter cannot be explained by the water content, analogous to our findings in cerebral edema, since in normal tissue the water content of the grey matter is on average 18.2% greater than that of white matter. The greater regional blood volume, the higher structural specific gravity of the grey matter and the myelin content in the fiber structures of the white matter are given as further reasons for the difference in X-ray absorption [11, 13, 17, 38, 52, 53, 72, 79].

Brooks et al. and Rieth et al. have related the Hounsfield units to the different chemical compositions of the grey and white matter. They see the reason for the different X-ray absorption as being that the grey matter contains 8% more oxygen atoms than the white matter, because of its higher water content (Table 4), and that the white matter contains about 8% more carbon atoms as a result of its higher lipid content (Table 4). Since the absorption of X-rays by a medium predominantly depends on the atomic number of the elements contained therein, the higher oxygen content (atomic number: 8, atomic weight: 16.0000) increases the X-ray absorption

Table 4. Content of hydrogen, carbon, nitrogen and oxygen in constituents of normal and edematous white matter. (From Rieth et al., 1980)

Substance	Total (%)	H (%)	C (%)	N (%)	O (%)	
Proteins	11.29	0.82	6.24	1.65	2.58	Normal white matter
Lipids	16.06	1.78	11.56	0.23	2.20	
Electrolytes	1.05	–	–	–	0.30	
Water	71.60	7.96	–	–	63.64	
Total	100.00	10.56	17.80	1.88	68.72	
Proteins	7.90	0.57	4.37	1.15	1.81	Edematous white matter
Lipids	11.23	1.24	8.08	0.16	1.54	
Electrolytes	1.17	–	–	–	0.334	
Water	79.70	8.86	–	–	70.84	
Total	100.00	10.67	12.45 △7.71	1.31	74.524 △7.74	

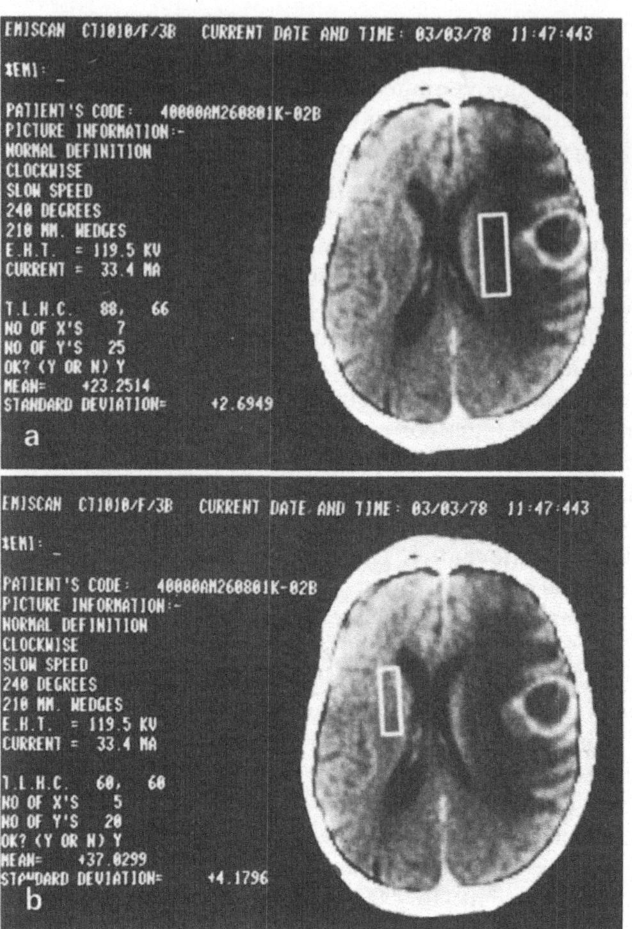

Fig. 1. a Area of measurement in a representative field containing edema. Mean absorption: +23.25 HU. **b** Area of measurement in the white substance of the control hemisphere. Mean absorption: +37.2 HU

in the grey matter. The 8% lower oxygen content in the white matter and the approximately 8% higher carbon content (atomic number: 6, atomic weight: 12.010) reduce the X-ray absorption in the cerebral tissue of the white matter.

Since the white matter, with darker shades of grey, stands out from the tissue areas of the grey matter, it is necessary to know the digital absorption values for diagnosis of a perifocal cerebral edema, otherwise the characteristic appearance of the centrum ovale could be misinterpreted as edema in the white matter. The edema in the area surrounding a compressive lesion appears considerably darker than the surrounding white matter.

The mean Hounsfield units of a zone of perifocal edema differ significantly from the corresponding Hounsfield units in the opposite hemisphere (Figs. 1a, b).

In the computed tomogram, slight perifocal edema shows a definite boundary line between the edema zone and the unaffected white matter (Figs. 2a, b, c). The cor-

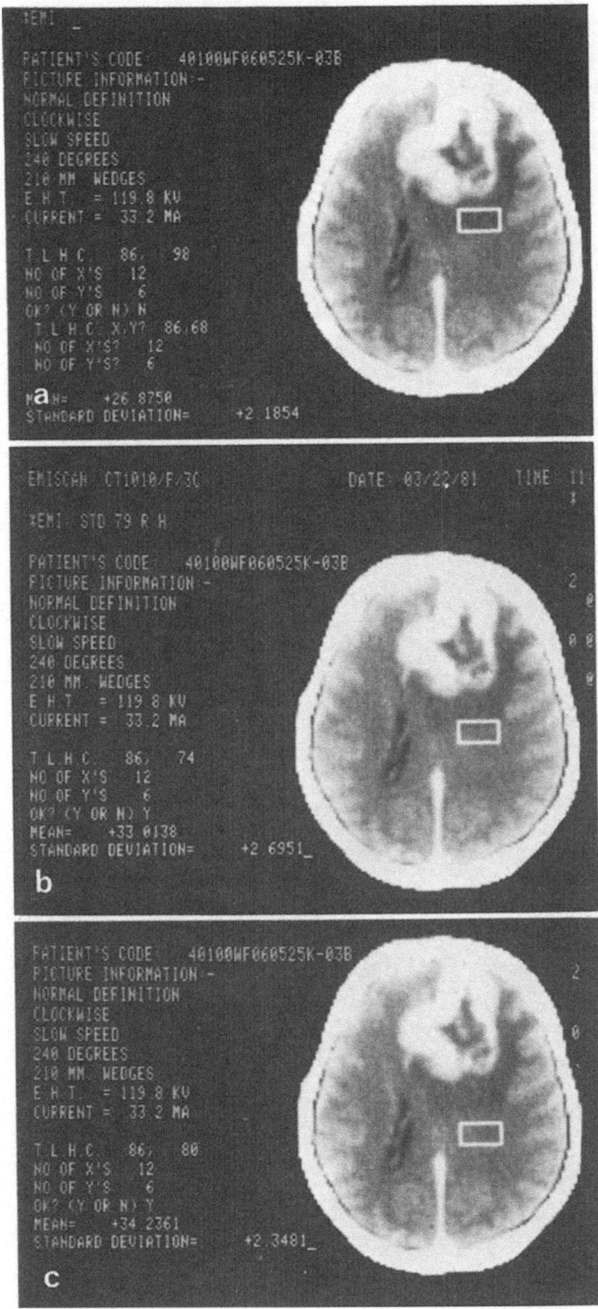

Fig. 2a–c. Areas of measurement, containing edematous zone and neighbouring white substance of a progressive distance from the tumor. The first area of measurement has an absorption of 26.87 HU. The following area with enlarged white substance has similar absorption values, which differ from that of the perifocal edema. The last area has a higher absorption (+40.55 HU) since the area contains cortical matter

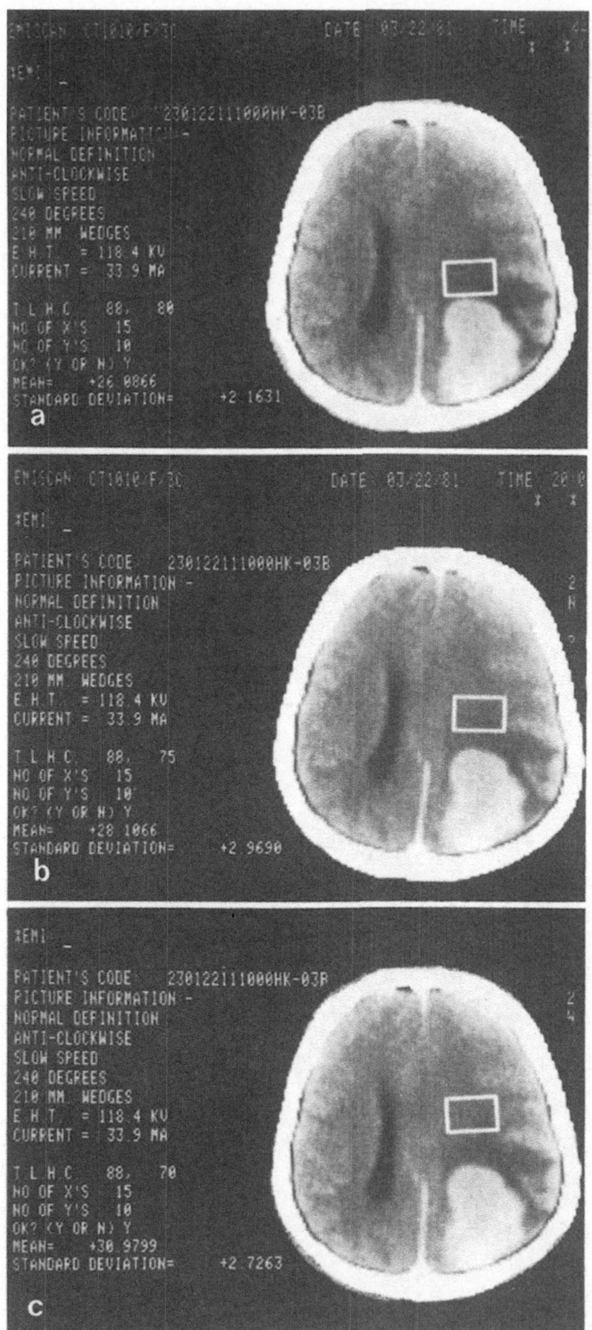

Fig. 3a–f. Areas of measurement in edematous zone and neighbouring white matter. The edema is not sharply demarcated from the white matter

PATIENT'S CODE 230122111000HK-03B
PICTURE INFORMATION -
NORMAL DEFINITION
ANTI-CLOCKWISE
SLOW SPEED
240 DEGREES
210 MM WEDGES
E H T = 118 4 KV
CURRENT = 33 9 MA
T L H C 88, 65
NO OF X'S 15
NO OF Y'S 10
OK? (Y OR N) Y
MEAN= +33 1599
STANDARD DEVIATION= +2 8567
d
PATIENT'S CODE 230122111000HK-03B
PICTURE INFORMATION -
NORMAL DEFINITION
ANTI-CLOCKWISE
SLOW SPEED
240 DEGREES
210 MM WEDGES
E H T = 118 4 KV
CURRENT = 33 9 MA
T L H C 88, 60
NO OF X'S 15
NO OF Y'S 10
OK? (Y OR N) Y
MEAN= +35 6666
STANDARD DEVIATION= +4 3060
e
PATIENT'S CODE 230122111000HK-03
PICTURE INFORMATION -
NORMAL DEFINITION
ANTI-CLOCKWISE
SLOW SPEED
240 DEGREES
210 MM WEDGES
E H T = 118 4 KV
CURRENT = 33 9 MA
T L H C 88, 55
NO OF X'S 15
NO OF Y'S 10
OK? (Y OR N) Y
MEAN= +37 1933
STANDARD DEVIATION= +4 0442
f

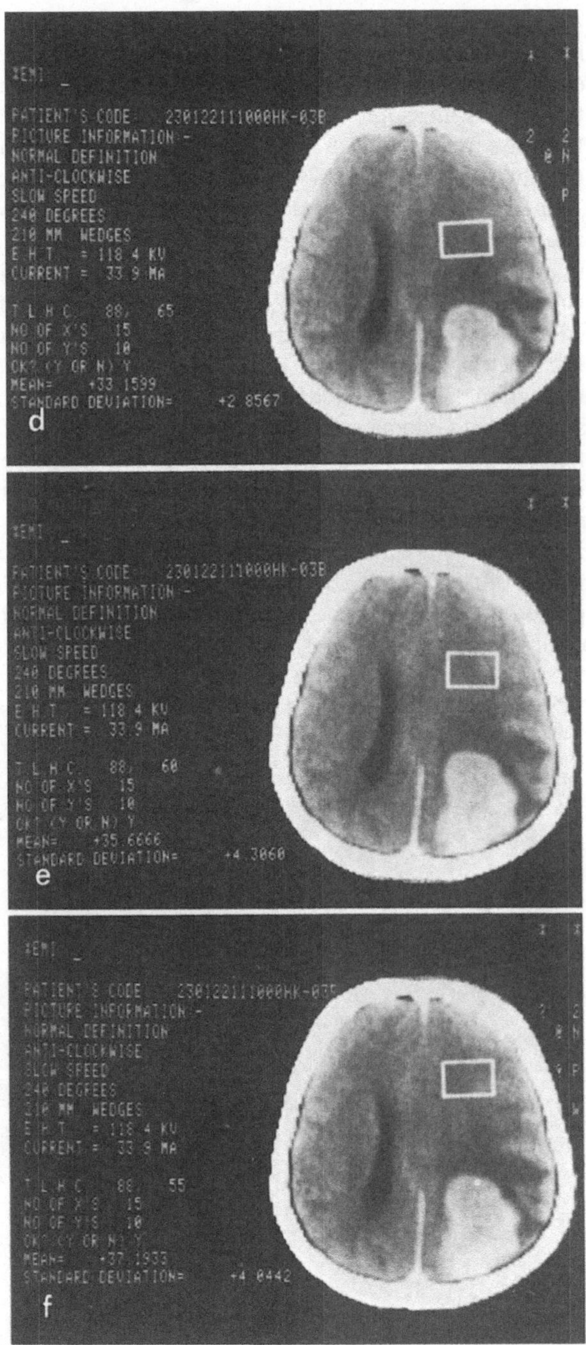

Fig. 3 d–f

responding absorption values of the adjacent regions demonstrate that the edema has not spread throughout the entire white matter. In most of the cases, the perifocal edema merges into the surrounding white matter. The average absorption values in the various measured regions of a zone of edema increase with increasing distances from the tumor (Figs. 3a–f). The lowest mean absorption value of a measurement field lying within an area of perifocal edema and directly adjacent to the tumor was 18.0 Hounsfield units in 180 cerebral tumor patients. Since we measured such low absorption values exclusively in cases of very extensive tumor edema, we assume that this absorption value is representative of maximum water absorption in the zone adjacent to the tumor. Additional absorption of water is evidently compensated by further spreading of the edema in the centrum ovale, or by edema absorption.

For the exact *localization of perifocal edema* in cerebral tumors in the computed tomogram, we compared the standard computed tomogram layers and the brain sections with edema symptoms by computed tomography. It was shown very clearly that the perifocal brain edema visible in the CT corresponds to the pattern of spread in the white matter [41]. The characteristic configurations which cerebral edema has in different tumor sites are thus explained.

In the case of a frontal tumor, the edema spreads in a fan-like manner in the white matter of the frontal lobe. The following characteristics are found, depending on the plane of section and the extent of the edema and independent of the underlying compressing lesion (Fig. 4).

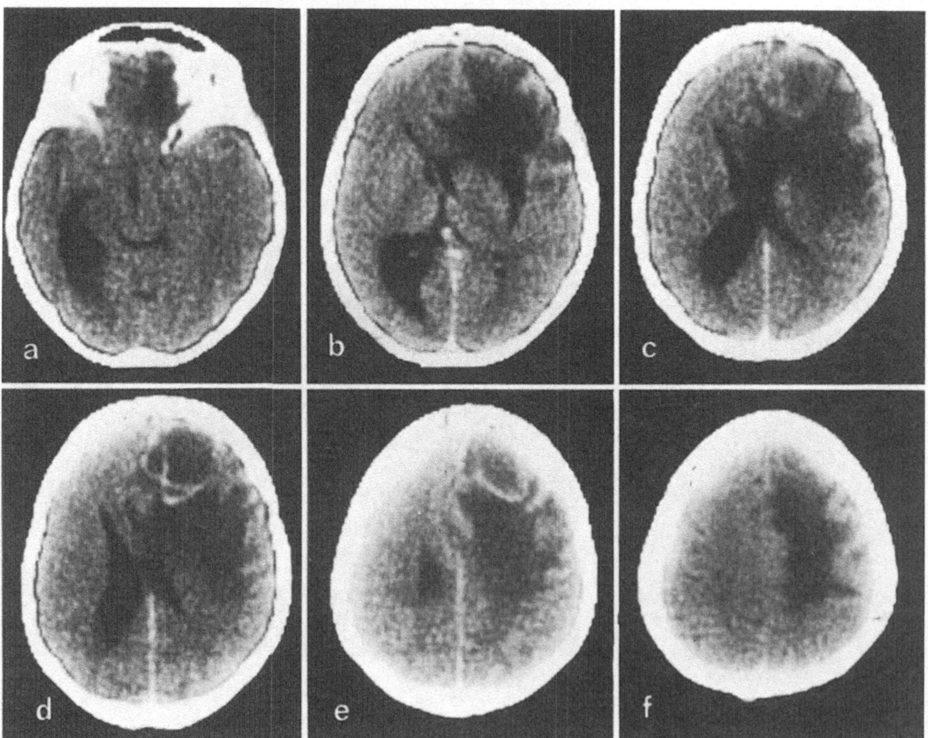

Fig. 4a–f. Extensive diffuse edema of grade III

The edema fans out from the center of the cerebral white matter forwards, sideways and backwards, and ends with wider or narrower branches in the superior frontal gyrus, in the middle frontal gyrus and in the inferior frontal gyrus. With the latter branch, the edema terminates opposite the lateral cerebral fissure. Of the two branches directed backwards, the lateral always terminates in the form of a funnel in an isthmus between the insular cortex and putamen of the lentiform nucleus. The computed tomograms give the impression that the edema cannot spread further between the structures of grey matter. The only way through for the edema (detectable by computed tomography) is the very narrow external capsule and the white of the insular cortex. The edema spreads, with expansion of the white matter in this isthmus, to the posterior end of the insular cortex only in cases where there is severe unilateral edema (Fig. 4). The medial of the two backward branches is directed either towards the third ventricle or to the tip of the anterior horn of the lateral ventricle on the same side, depending on the plane of section (Fig. 4). At higher planes of section (above the basal ganglia) the edema spreads unimpeded in the white matter of the frontal lobe and also penetrates – depending on the extent of the edema – that of the parietal lobe (Fig. 4). If expanding lesions are strictly localized frontally on one side, the edema only crosses the midline to the opposite side firstly if extensive edema from the frontal white matter has access to the corpus callosum and secondly if this access to the corpus callosum is not itself obstructed by the tumor. On the basis of our computed tomography investigations, spread of edema in the frontal white matter across the midline to the opposite side takes place only via the "bridge" of the anterior radiation of the corpus callosum ("forceps minor").

In the computed tomogram, *expanding lesions in the temporal region* are surrounded by zones of edema of characteristic configuration, depending on the site of the lesion within the temporal lobe and the extent of the edema. In our investigation of 602 meningiomas [34], temporal convexity meningiomas and lateral sphenoidal meningiomas showed the most extensive edema in this region; the edema of a sphenoidal meningioma will be described below as a typical example. Figure 5a shows the basal portion of a temporal edema. The zone of reduced density outlined in the manner of a map corresponds to the white matter of the basal temporal lobe. The layers directly above (Figs. 5b, c) show the edema with two foci. On the one hand, the edema spreads into the white matter of the frontal lobe, and on the other hand into the posterior portion of the temporal lobe. Three characteristic finger-like branches of edema can be seen extending from the center of the white matter of the posterior temporal region (Fig. 5b). The medial branch follows the posterior portion of the inner capsule forwards, and is bounded medially by the thalamus and laterally by the lentiform nucleus (pallidum). The middle branch extends forwards in the external capsule and the white matter of the insular cortex, between this and the lentiform nucleus. The lateral branch of the edema corresponds to the white centrum of the temporal lobe. This configuration is approximately maintained at the next higher level (Fig. 5c), but the spread of the edema into the white matter, with recesses in all structures of grey matter, is substantially more obvious. In particular, the middle branch of the edema marks the adjacent regions of grey matter, medially the lentiform nucleus and laterally the insular cortex and the cortex band of the superior temporal gyrus, which is seen to be clearly separated from the insula by the lateral cerebral fissure. A narrow strip of increased density can be seen in

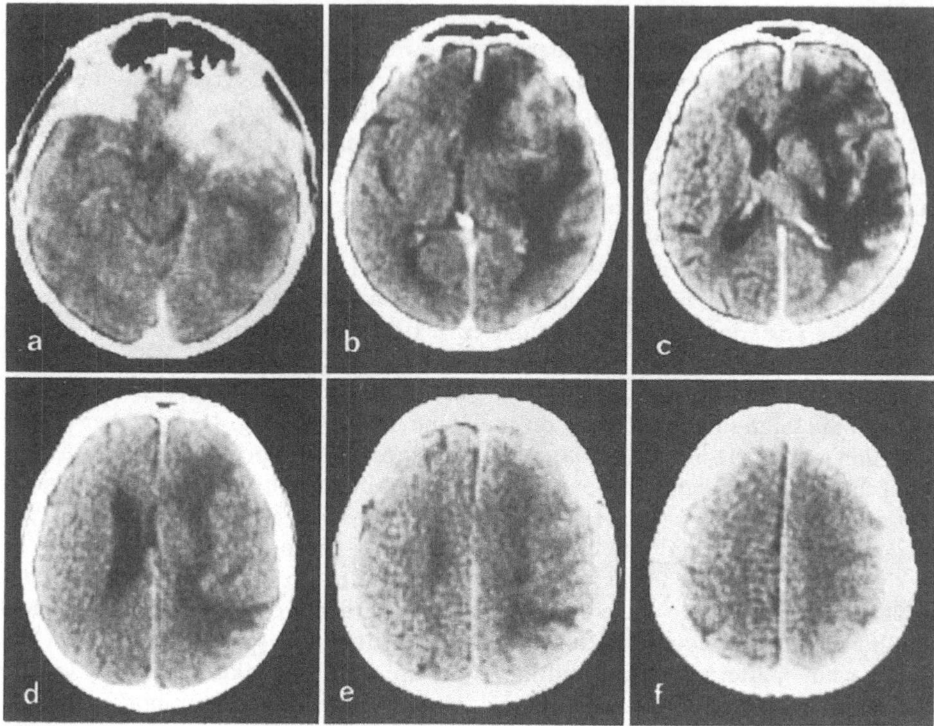

Fig. 5a–f. Excensive perifocal edema due to a temporal space-occupying lesion. The finger type edema reaches the basal ganglia and the Sylvian fissure (**b, c**). In the following sections the edema reaches the white matter of the parietal lobe

the middle branch, and this strip again seems to be recessed by the edema and corresponds to the claustrum. In an occipital direction, the edema still appears in the adjacent parts of white matter of the occipital lobe, with recesses in the cortical band. As the next higher planes of section show, the spread of edema of a temporal lesion extends into the parietal region under certain circumstances. In Figure 10d, the edema passes through the structures of white matter between the fissure of Sylvius and the top parts of the basal ganglia, and spreads out in the white matter of the frontal and occipital lobes.

Extensive perifocal edema from temporal lesions in the region of the fissure of Sylvius have an appearance in the computed tomogram as regards their spread in a longitudinal direction similar to the edema of a sphenoidal meningioma described above. However, their transverse spread differs. This example of a ring-shaped metastasis (Figs. 6a–d) shows how the edema has penetrated the white matter of the temporal lobe in the region of the fissure of Sylvius (superior temporal gyrus) from a lateral direction, i.e. from the side of the tumor, and has progressed frontally and occipitally on the other side of the cortical band of the insula in its white matter and in the external capsule (Fig. 6a). The adjacent layers, towards the vertex, show a broad band of edema temporoparietally in the centrum ovale, with cone-shaped recesses in the cortical band.

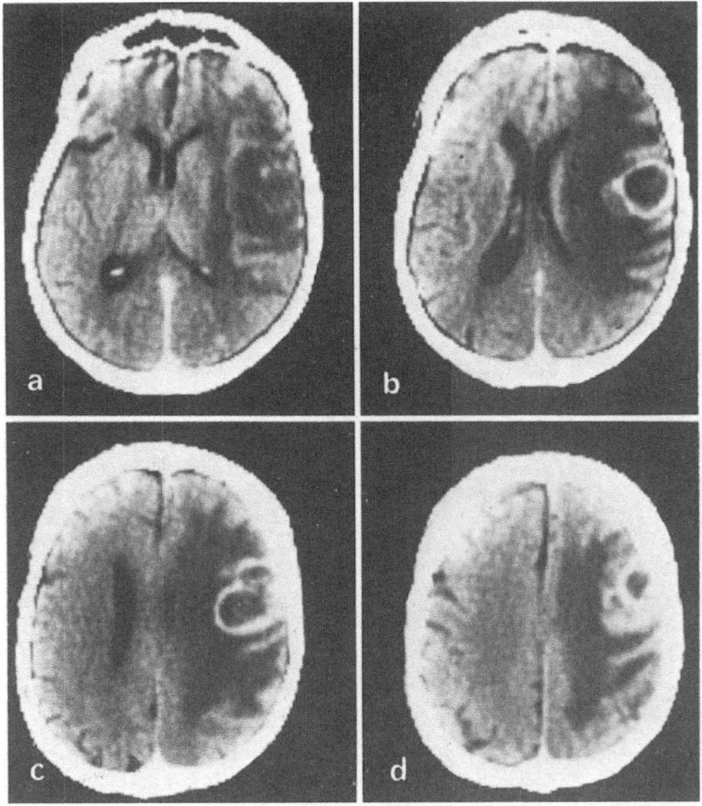

Fig. 6a–d. Perifocal edema *due to a metastasis* in the region of the Sylvian fissure. The edema reaches the external capsule and spreads to the occipital and frontal regions

Occipital Expanding Lesions

In the computed tomogram, occipital expanding lesions are surrounded by perifocal edema which has a similar pattern of spread to the edema of temporal lesions. The dark zones of reduced density are found in the white matter of the occipital lobe, depending on the site of the expanding lesion in the occipital lobe and of the extent of the edema (Fig. 7). From here, the edema extends on the one hand frontally into the medullary portions of the temporal lobe and the fibrous structures of the internal and external capsule (Fig. 7), and on the other hand into the medullary center of the parietal lobe. No edema can be detected by computed tomography in the cerebral tissue portions of grey matter, the cortical stribs, the thalamus and the lentiform nucleus. These structures, and the fissure of Sylvius, represent the boundaries of the perifocal edema in the computed tomogram. As is the case in the region of the anterior radiation of the corpus callosum, we have also observed spread of the edema across the midline to the opposite side through the posterior radiation of the corpus callosum ("forceps major") (Figs. 7a–c). Temporo-occipital expanding lesions which themselves largely occupy the medullary center of the occipital lobe,

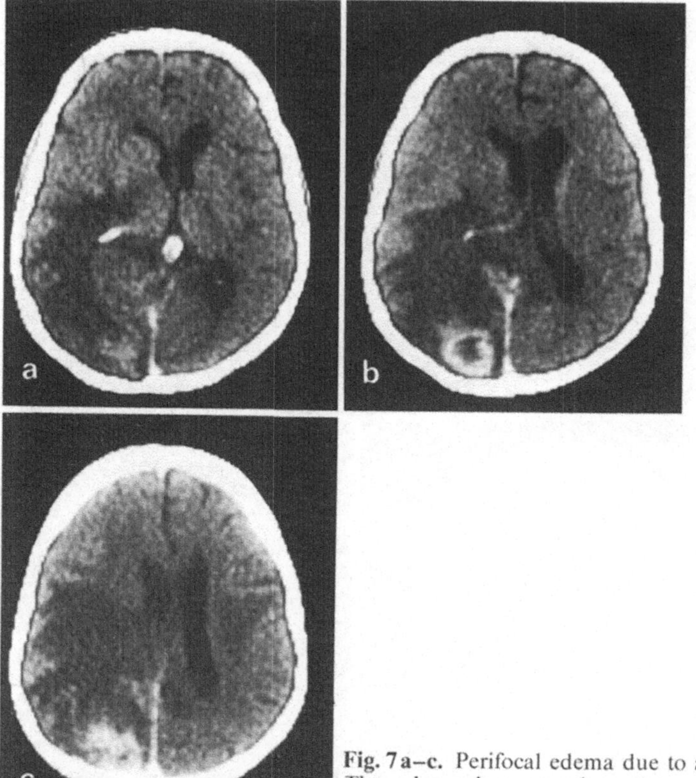

Fig. 7a–c. Perifocal edema due to an occipital metastasis. The edema has spread to the contralateral hemisphere via the posterior radiation of the corpus callosum

are restricted medially by the thalamus and extend fronto-laterally up to the fissure of Sylvius and show a spread of edema only along the white structures in the region of the internal capsule and the external capsule. In the case shown in Fig. 18, the edema within the grossly swollen internal capsule extends forwards up to the anterior horn of the right lateral ventricle. No spread of edema in a frontal direction can be detected beyond the anterior horn of the lateral ventricle.

In the computed tomogram, *the perifocal edema of expanding lesions in the parietal region* is shown as a zone of reduced density which varies in size and is divided into many parts. An example of extensive perifocal edema is shown in Fig. 8, in a case of a right parietal metastasis from a bronchial carcinoma. In the ventricular plane of section (Fig. 8 b), the edema is restricted medially by the lateral ventricle. In the higher layers (Figs. 8 c, d), the edema extends medially up to the cortical strip in the region of the margin of the mantle. The division of the edema zone in all the supraventricular layers corresponds to the distribution pattern of the white matter which is most prominent in the centrum ovale. The strip-like branches of the cerebral white matter which protrude into the tips of the cerebral convolutions appear as though outlined by the edema. Perifocal edema which extends into the lower layers from the parietal region not only continues medial to the fissure of Sylvius into the white matter of the temporal lobe and into the internal and ex-

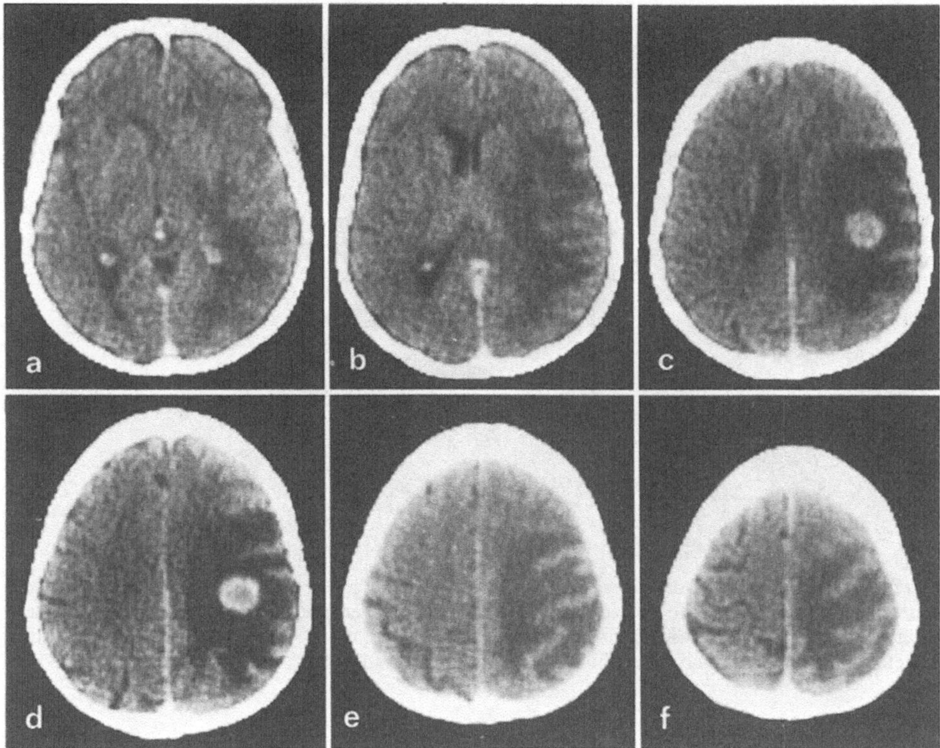

Fig. 8a–f. Extensive edema (grade III) due to a metastasis in the parietal lobe. The cortical layers are not affected, which leads to a comb-like appearance of the edema (**c, d**)

ternal capsule, but also continues laterally from the fissure into the white matter of the parietal and frontal cortex. On the basis of our investigations by computed tomography, it can be said that the spread of edema from the cranial to the caudal region always affects in addition the white matter of the strip of parietal cortex above and along the fissure of Sylvius. In contrast, we have observed that edema which spreads from the temporal or occipital region cranially can leave recesses in the frontal and parietal parts of the parenchyma lined by the fissure of Sylvius.

If these various computed tomographical edema images are represented on a frontal section through the brain at the level of the anterior pole of the temporal lobe (Fig. 9), it then becomes clear why these images are formed in the computed tomogram. A localized edema in the temporal or occipital lobes, with a tendency to extend cranially (Fig. 9, right-hand half of the picture) can reach the white matter below the lateral cerebral fissure and can continue medial to the fissure of Sylvius, along the external capsule and the white of the insular cortex upwards into the parietal lobe. On the basis of our investigations, the edema evidently does not spread laterally or diagonally downwards into the white matter of the parietal lobe above the lateral cerebral fissure. Edema which spreads caudally from the parietal region behaves conversely (Fig. 9 left). The white matter above the lateral cerebral fissure is reached by the edema, which can in turn spread medial to the fissure of Sylvius

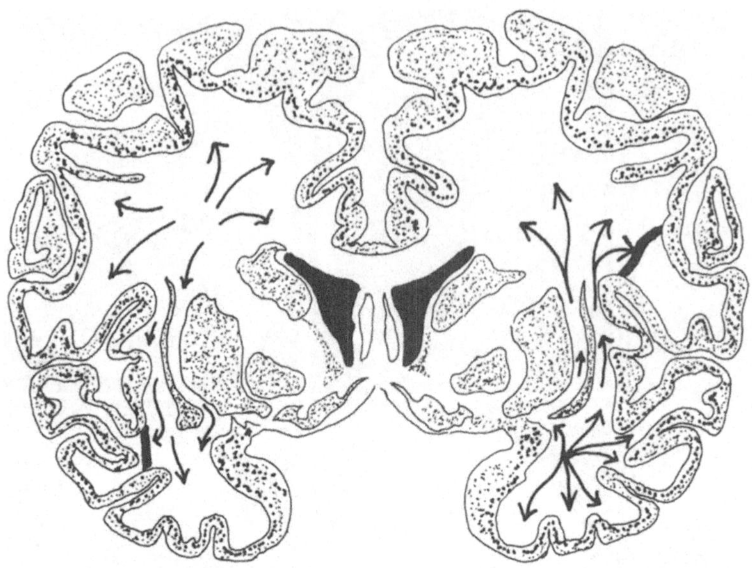

Fig. 9. Schematic representation of a coronal section at the level of the anterior part of the ventricles. On the right side the edema spreads from the temporal lobe to the vertex. Edema located above the insular cortex never spreads in a caudal direction (right-sided arrow) to the parietal white matter. In contrast the parietal edema spreads above the insular cortex

downwards or caudally, but does not continue into the temporal or frontal lobe below the fissure. Very extensive perifocal edema in parietal lesions can penetrate the entire centrum ovale, which is as a rule thereby very broadened or expanded, from front to back.

Our examinations of the various appearances of edema in expanding lesions in the computed tomogram, in comparison with normal intracranial structures in horizontal brain sections enable us to draw the following conclusions:

a) Perifocal vasogenic edema of expanding lesions can always be detected in the white matter in the computed tomogram, independently of its site. The topography of the cerebral white matter and of the other fibrous tissue is thus responsible for the appearances produced by perifocal edema in the computed tomogram.
b) Of the perifocal edemas visible in the computed tomogram, the entire cortical grey matter and the grey matter of the basal ganglia as a rule remain recessed.
c) In almost all cases, contact can be detected between the ramifications of the edema and the internal and external subarachnoid spaces, independent of the site of the perifocal cerebral edema.

Computed tomographical detection of perifocal cerebral edema in the white matter corresponds to experience gained in animal experiments with vasogenic cerebral edema which spreads almost exclusively in the extracellular spaces of the white matter [7, 9, 15, 19, 25, 26, 60, 65–70, 75].

The perifocal edema of implanted rat gliomas observed in cats by Hossmann et al. [27] was found exclusively in the white matter.

Compared with these numerous experimental studies of vasogenic cerebral edema carried out on animals, there have been only relatively few studies concerning quantitative and qualitative investigations of vasogenic cerebral edema in humans. Both electron microscope studies [81] and biochemical analyses of cerebral tissue samples which have been obtained during neurosurgical operations from edema zones close to tumors [40, 47, 48, 65, 66, 77] show, in agreement with each other, that vasogenic edema can chiefly be detected in the white matter, since the increase in water content in the grey matter is less than that in the white matter (Table 5). When comparing normal human cerebral tissue with that which has undergone edematous change, however, all the authors refer to the normal values published by Yates et al. [86]. On the basis of the compilation in Table 5, the average increase in water in the white matter of 98 patients with cerebral tumors is 10.5%, based on a normal value of 69.1% [86]. In contrast, the water content in the grey matter has increased on average only by 0.7%. From these quantitative values, it can be said that the detection of peritumoral cerebral edema predominantly in the white matter by computed tomography corresponds to the underlying differing increases in water content in the grey matter and in the white matter. The computed tomography findings could give the impression that perifocal cerebral tumor edema is exclusively a phenomenon of the white matter, since edema-related reductions in density in parts of the grey matter are only rarely seen.

The explanation for this is the relatively low increase in water content in the grey matter (Table 5), which cannot be recognized because of the limited power of density-resolution of the CT apparatus. Only in 39 (1.1%) out of 3,750 patients with cerebral tumors did we find reductions in density in areas of grey matter adjacent to the tumor, which were detectable by computed tomography. These patients were suffering from glioblastomas (22 cases) and metastases (17 cases), which were located either in the posterior part of the temporal lobe or in the temporo-occipital transition area (Fig. 10). All the tumors were immediately adjacent to the thalamus, which had lower absorption values in comparison with the opposite side. On the basis of our investigations, development of edema in the grey matter which can be detected by computed tomography, occurs only in cases of glioblastoma and cerebral metastases which are located in the immediate neighborhood of the thalamus or the lentiform nucleus.

Table 5. Water content in tissue samples from peritumoral zones of edema in brain tumors

	Water content in %	
	White matter	Grey matter
Schmiedek (1972)	79.03 ($n=25$)	81.94 ($n=27$)
Reulen (1972)	79.00 ($n=18$)	81.00 ($n=18$)
Meinig (1976)	79.90 ($n=31$)	81.60 ($n=31$)
Lanksch (1976)	78.78 ($n=15$)	83.70 ($n=15$)
Lanksch (1977)	81.36 ($n=9$)	83.77 ($n=9$)
Mean value:	$\bar{x}=79.61$	$\bar{x}=82.38$
Normal value Yates (1975)	69.10	81.70
Difference	△ *10.51*	△ *0.68*

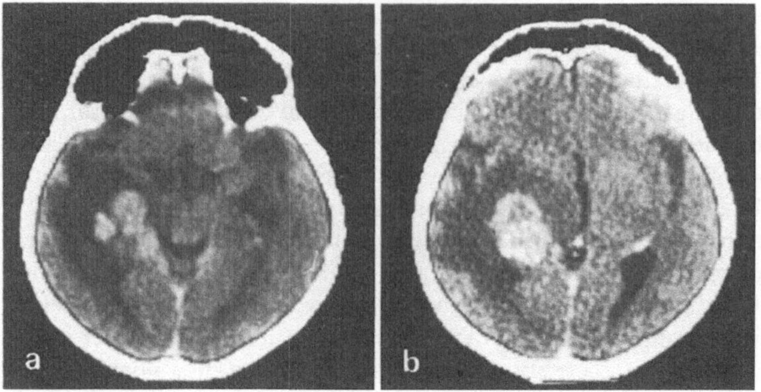

Fig. 10a, b. Perifocal edema due to a left-sided temporal metastasis, reaching not only the temporo-occipital white matter but also the thalamus

Especially in cases of tumor edema in the frontal white matter we have observed that the edema frequently is adjacent to the anterior horn of the lateral ventricle (Figs. 11, 12). Expanding lesions in the temporal and occipital regions also show edema branches which are in contact with the anterior horn if this part of the ventricle is the only part which can be reached, i.e. if the route the edema takes in spreading through the white matter to the next closest part of the lateral ventricle is

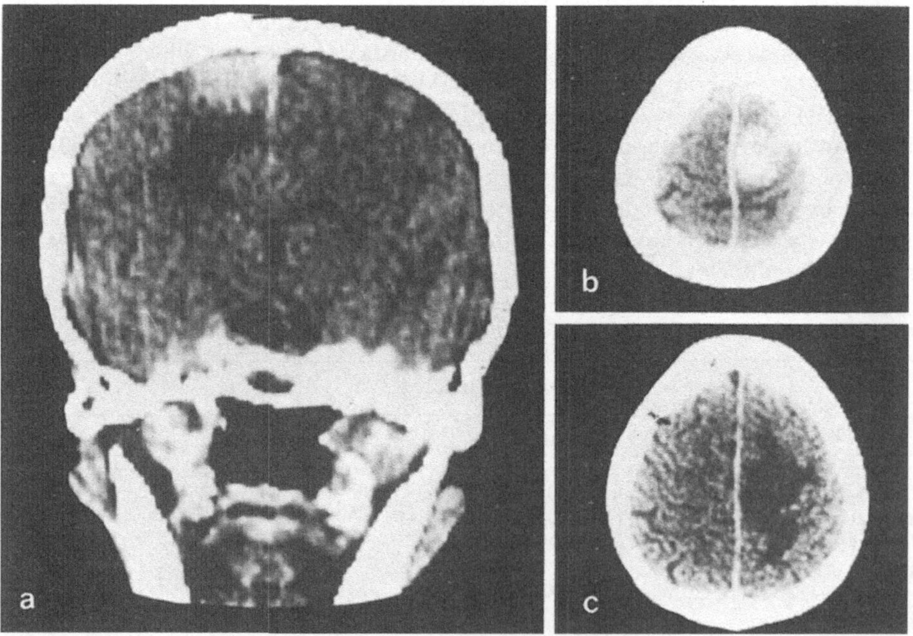

Fig. 11a–c. Perifocal edema caused by a right-sided parasagittal meningioma. The edema has spread to the frontal region (**c**) and comes into contact with the frontal horn of the lateral ventricle

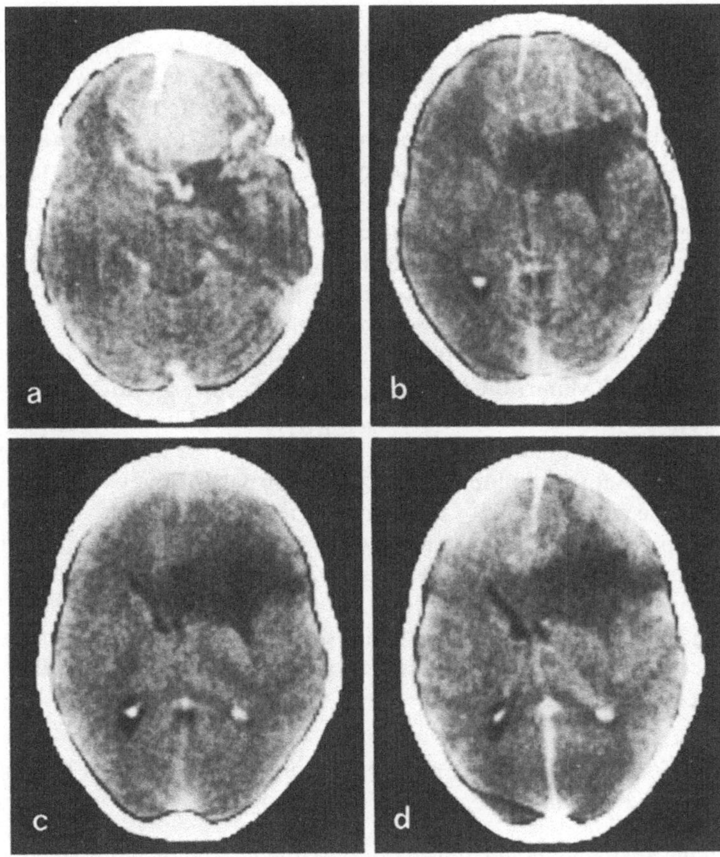

Fig. 12a–d. Frontobasal meningioma with typical pattern of perifocal edema, reaching the ventricular system

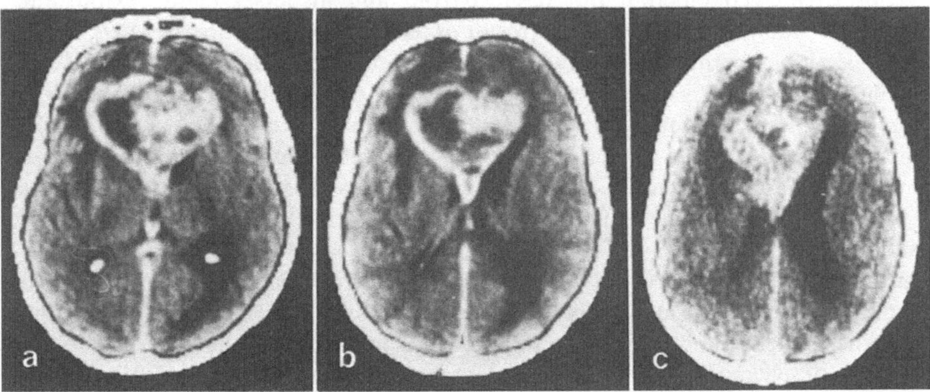

Fig. 13a–c. Bifrontal ("butterfly") glioblastoma limited on the right side by the lateral ventricle and markedly compressed on the left side by the frontal aspect of the lateral ventricle and the cella media. A small amount of edema can be seen on the left side in the white matter

blocked by the tumor itself. In our opinion, these observations confirm the experimental results obtained by Reulen et al. [65, 66, 68], who detected, in cases of edema after cold lesions of the frontal cortex, a bulk flow of the edema fluid from the site of the lesion through the white matter into the ventricle. These authors consider that the transport of the edema fluid from the white matter via the ependyma into the ventricle fluid is an important, if not the most important, mechanism of absorption of the vasogenic edema. So-called butterfly gliomas which extend from the anterior or posterior end of the corpus callosum largely symmetrically between the lateral ventricles and in front or behind these bilaterally into the white matter of the hemispheres show edema images in the computed tomogram which confirm the above mentioned edema absorption mechanism. Figure 13 shows a butterfly glioblastoma in the anterior part of the corpus callosum. The tumor has obstructed the foramen of Monro on the right side, with corresponding expansion of the lateral ventricle. On the left side, the anterior horn is almost completely obliterated. In the computed tomogram, the spread of edema can be recognized only on the left side in the adjacent frontal lobe and the anterior part of the external capsule. On the right side, the entire spread of the tumor is along the medial wall of the lateral ventricle. No spread of edema, which would be possible to the right frontally into the white matter, can be detected; the edema fluid is evidently drained directly via the ependyma of the ventricular wall into the CSF pathways.

Since computed tomography cannot detect dynamic processes but only morphological changes, we view with reservation these statements regarding dynamic processes in cerebral edema.

The Effect of an Iodine-Containing Contrast Medium on Perifocal Cerebral Edema as seen in the Computed Tomogram

In the analogue image, it was not possible to recognize any change in the absorption figures in the perifocal edema either in the tumors with contrast intensification or in the tumors which remained unchanged in the computed tomogram after injection of a contrast medium. Since the contrast medium leaves the intravascular space in the case of a damaged blood/tumor tissue barrier and disperses in the extracellular space of the tumor parenchyma as a result of its hydrophilic properties [39], there is the question of whether the contrast medium can also pass the blood-brain barrier, the function of which is demonstrably disturbed when a vasogenic cerebral edema is present [35]. Experimental studies carried out on animals to the neurotoxicity of iodine-containing contrast media have shown that such contrast media damage the function of the blood-brain barrier and can also pass through the blood-brain barrier, depending on their chemical structure, iodine content and osmolality and the amount administered [37, 49, 76, 82].

This pharmacokinetic aspect of contrast medium distribution in the cerebral parenchyma can be investigated only to a limited extent by computed tomography. Nevertheless, it seemed to us to be important to test whether the absorption values of areas of edema in the computed tomogram change after intravenous administration of an iodine-containing contrast medium.

Such a measurement procedure will be demonstrated using as an example an olfactory nerve meningioma, which appears with isodense absorption values in

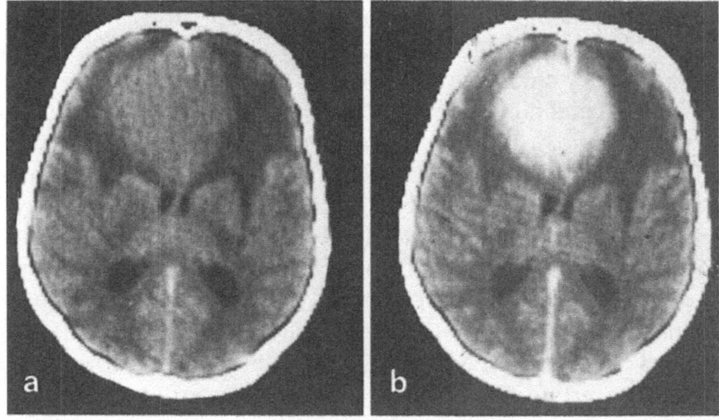

Fig. 14a, b. Olfactory groove meningioma with bilateral edema. Contrast medium does not change the absorption values in the edema, as it does in the tumour tissue

the plain CT (Fig. 14). After administration of the contrast medium, the tumor manifests itself with significantly increased density values. The average absorption value in the plain CT of 43.63 HU is increased to 68.87 by administration of the contrast medium. In contrast, the average absorption value in the measurement field of the perifocal edema of 26.28 HU in the plain CT is increased by 0.74 HU to 27.02 HU after administration of the contrast medium. This increase in density values cannot be found in the analogue image (Fig. 14). Since the margin of error in the measurement system is about 0.9 HU, the increase in the mean absorption value in the perifocal edema after administration of the contrast medium is restricted to one Hounsfield unit.

The average absorption values in the edema zones of 105 patients ranged from 18.8 HU to 29.0 HU. After administration of a contrast medium (a 66% solution of the meglumine salt of ioxitalamic acid – Telebrix 300^{R} –; 1 ml/kg of body weight, intravenously as a bolus), the absorption values in the corresponding edema zones varied from 19.0 HU to 29.0 HU, with a mean value of 22.3 HU. The absorption values measured by us in the zones of edema before and after administration of the contrast medium showed no significant difference, even when the second measurement was made only 30–40 minutes after administration of the contrast medium. With the limited density-resolution power of this generation of instruments, the permeation of iodine-containing contrast medium from the intravascular space into the extracellular space of the edematous parenchyma can be neither detected nor excluded. For the present state of the technique, it can only be said that administration of a contrast medium has no effect which can be detected by computed tomography on the absorption values in the perifocal zones of edema. This means that in the boundary region between tumor and perifocal edema, only the absorption values of the tumor tissue and not those of the zone of edema change after administration of contrast medium, which in most cases enables clear demarcation between the marginal zone, between the tumor and the perifocal edema in the analogue image obtained by computed tomography.

Frequency and Spread of Perifocal Edema in Cases of Cerebral Tumor

The frequency and spread of perifocal cerebral edema was determined in 3,750 patients with cerebral tumors. The large number of patients in this investigation series arises from a joint study carried out by the three CT study groups at the Neurosurgical University Clinics in Munich and Berlin (Charlottenburg Clinic) and in the Neuroradiological Department of the Neurosurgical University Clinic in Mainz [34]. The 3750 cerebral tumors evaluated by computed tomography are compiled in Table 6 according to their histological classification. With the exception of the tumor groups "other cerebral tumors" and "cerebral tumors of unknown histology", the diagnosis was made according to the cerebral tumor classification of the WHO. Tumors which occurred rarely and in a number too low for them to be shown individually in our series are classified in the group "other cerebral tumors". The group "cerebral tumors of unknown histology" comprises those cerebral tumors on which no histological examination could be carried out because they were inoperable.

As well as the most important histological diagnoses, Table 6 also summarizes the frequency and extent of perifocal edema in 3,750 cerebral tumors. The varying extent of perifocal edema was classified into three degrees [41]; degree I edema: perifocal edema limbus up to 2 cm wide; degree II edema: perifocal edema which occupies up to half of one hemisphere; degree III edema: perifocal edema which occupies more than half of one hemisphere. The complete evaluation shows that of 3,750 intracranial tumors, 1,970 (52.5%) show a perifocal cerebral edema in the computed tomogram. Of these 1,970 intracranial tumors, 759 (38.5%) were surrounded by a degree I edema, 953 (48.4%) were surrounded by a degree II edema and 258 (13.1%) were surrounded by a degree III edema. Since a degree III edema is recorded only in 13.1% of all the cases, and thus relatively rarely, we have added together the cases with degree II and degree III edema in each tumor group. The ratio of degree II and III edemas to degree I edemas in each tumor group is shown in Table 7. The quotient given by the ratio of 1,211 degree II and III edemas to 759 degree I edemas in all the 3,750 cerebral tumors is 1.6. However, this quotient is greater than 1 in only six out of all the 18 tumor groups. The quotient is 3.1 for glioblastomas, 1.9 for metastases, 1.2 for malignant lymphomas, 1.1 for grade III astrocytomas, 1.5 for meningiomas and also 1.5 for the group "other cerebral tumors". The remaining 12 tumor groups have a degree II + III/degree I quotient of less than 1.0, i.e. the grade I edema predominates in these tumor groups.

If the tumor groups with an edema degree quotient of more than 1.0 are summarized separately (without taking into consideration the collective group "other cerebral tumors"), these 2,107 cerebral tumors have 550 with degree I edema and 1,122 with degree II and III edema give a quotient of 2.0. This means that the tumors which most frequently show cerebral edema (on average 79.3%) also usually show degree II and III edema in the computed tomogram. With the exception of the meningiomas, the tumors (glioblastomas, metastases, malignant lymphomas and degree III astrocytomas) are classified as malignant.

On the other hand, our investigations show that the intracranial tumors which have only an average edema frequency of 33% (without taking into consideration the dysontogenetic processes, the cerebral tumors of unknown histology, the degree II

Table 6. Frequency and spread of the perifocal brain edema in 3,750 brain tumors

Type diagnosis	No. of patients	Total number	Perifocal edema		
			Degree I	Degree II	Grade III
Astrocytoma (degree II)	153	3 (2.0%)	2 (66.7%)	1 (33.3%)	–
Astrocytoma (degree III)	157	106 (67.5%)	51 (48.0%)	47 (44.5%)	8 (7.5%)
Oligodendroglioma	174	66 (38.0%)	38 (57.6%)	25 (37.9%)	3 (4.5%)
Glioblastoma	711	652 (92.0%)	160 (24.5%)	376 (57.6%)	116 (17.8%)
Pilocytic astrocytoma	112	28 (25.0%)	26 (93.0%)	2 (7.0%)	–
Ependymoma	54	23 (42.6%)	14 (61.0%)	6 (26.0%)	3 (13.0%)
Medulloblastoma	67	31 (46.3%)	28 (90.3%)	3 (9.7%)	–
Malignant lymphosarcomas	62	45 (72.6%)	20 (44.0%)	22 (49.0%)	3 (7.0%)
Plexus papilloma	14	6 (42.8%)	4 (66.0%)	1 (17.0%)	1 (17.0%)
Meningioma	602	369 (61.3%)	147 (40.0%)	181 (49.0%)	41 (11.0%)
Neurinoma	196	53 (27.0%)	47 (88.7%)	5 (9.4%)	1 (1.9%)
Pituitary adenoma	377	5 (1.3%)	5 (100%)	–	–
Hemangioblastoma	41	10 (24.4%)	9 (90.0%)	1 (10.0%)	–
Craniopharyngioma	81	1 (1.2%)	1 (100%)	–	–
Epidermoid-dermoid teratoma	36	2 (5.5%)	2 (100%)	–	–
Other brain tumors	192	38 (19.8%)	15 (39.5%)	17 (44.7%)	6 (15.8%)
Brain metastases	575	500 (87.0%)	172 (34.4%)	253 (50.6%)	75 (15.0%)
Brain tumors of unknown histology	146	32 (22.0%)	18 (56.2%)	13 (40.6%)	1 (3.2%)
Total	3,750	1,970 (52.5%)	759 (38.5%)	953 (48.4%)	258 (13.1%)

Table 7. Ratio of edema degree II + III to edema degree I in 3,750 intracranial tumors

Type of tumor	No.	Edema degree I	Edema degree II + III	Ratio II + III/I
Glioblastoma	711	160	492	3.1
Metastases	575	172	328	1.9
Malignant lymphoma	62	20	25	1.2
Astrocytoma III	157	51	55	1.1
Meningioma	602	147	222	1.5
Medulloblastoma	67	28	3	0.1
Plexus papilloma	14	4	2	0.5
Ependymoma	54	14	9	0.6
Oligodendroglioma	174	38	28	0.7
Neurinoma	196	47	6	0.1
Pilocytic astrocytoma	112	26	2	0.1
Hemangioblastoma	41	9	1	0.1
Brain tumors of unknown histology	146	18	14	0.7
Other brain tumors	192	15	23	1.5
Epidermoid-dermoid teratoma	36	2	–	–
Astrocytoma II	153	2	1	0.5
Pituitary adenoma	377	5	–	–
Craniopharyngioma	81	1	–	–
Total	3,750	759	1,211	1.6

astrocytomas (in which tumor tissue and edema cannot be differentiated because of their identical absorption values) and pituitary adenomas) chiefly show degree I edema in the computed tomogram.

Moreover, statistical analysis (chi-square test) of the edema frequency in 3,750 intracranial tumors showed, at a high level of significance, that glioblastomas and cerebral metastases more frequently showed cerebral edema in the computed tomogram than the other tumors. In contrast, oligodendrogliomas, neurinomas, pilocytic astrocytomas and hemangioblastomas are, at a high level of significance, more rarely accompanied by edema in the computed tomogram than the other intracranial tumors.

Characteristic Findings on Investigation of Intracranial Tumors

In the following, only those groups of tumors will be presented in which characteristic findings in respect of the diagnosis of cerebral edema are found in the computed tomogram.

Astrocytomas II (fibrillar and protoplasmic A.) appear in the computed tomogram uniformly as localized circular or oval (Fig. 15), occasionally map-like zones of reduced density. The average absorption values of 22 HU correspond to those of brain edema. The high water content of these tumors of 80–82% [46], and their poor vascularization [30] are probably responsible for the low absorption values in the

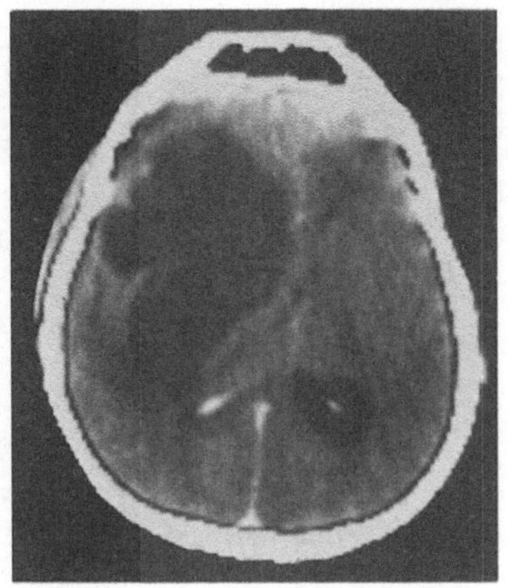

Fig. 15. Fronto-temporal astrocytoma grade II with hypodense areas without any increase of absorption after administration of contrast medium

computed tomogram. As a result of the poor vascularization, no contrast intensification of the tumor tissue can be obtained by means of a contrast medium. Demarcation of the tumor from any perifocal edema is thus not possible. The density resolving power of the CT instruments of the 3rd generation is not sufficient to establish whether grade II astrocytomas develop perifocal edema or not.

Anaplastic astrocytomas, which show a contrast intensification in the computed tomogram after administration of contrast medium, are either predominantly cystic or predominantly solid tumors. The cystic tumors are distinguished in the computed tomogram by a relatively sharp boundary of the areas of the tumor with decreased density. The take-up of contrast medium occurs in the form of a ring, as a more or less complete outline of the cystic tumor. Among the predominantly solid anaplastic tumors, some appear in the plain CT like cystic astrocytomas, but take up contrast medium in the area of the tumor or on the interface with normal brain tissue; this always produces a demarcation between tumor and perifocal edema (Fig. 16).

Very large anaplastic astrocytomas occasionally present in the computed tomogram without any perifocal edema. The lack of cerebral edema is understandable after an

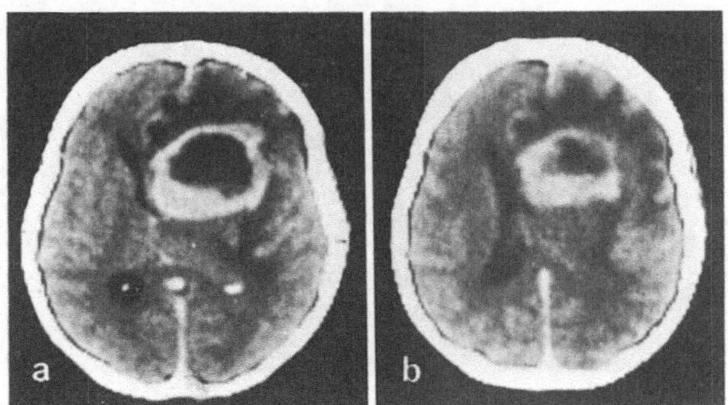

Fig. 16 a, b. Right frontal anaplastic astrocytoma with edema spreading only in a frontal direction. In the dorsal part of the tumor edema can spread only to the internal and external capsule. Slight edema can be seen in the Sylvian fissure

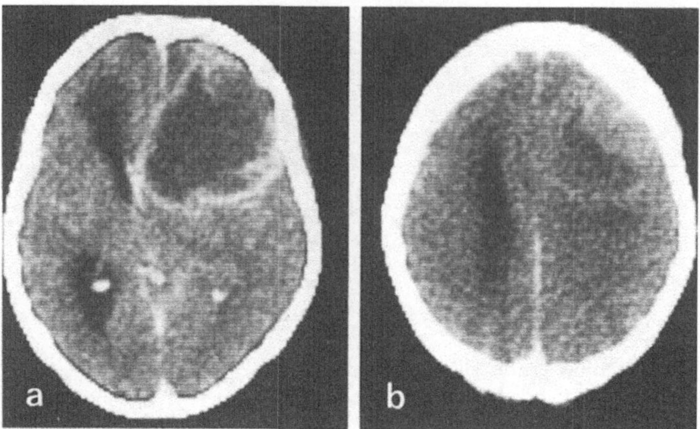

Fig. 17 a, b. Anaplastic astrocytoma, right fronto-parietal. Spread of the edema is possible only into the parietal white matter, since the basal ganglia and Sylvian fissure only allow it to spread into this area

exact analysis of the image. If the tumor spreads out so that its boundary coincides with that of the cerebral lobe affected, or if the tumor is bounded by grey matter structures, e.g. the basal ganglia, or the fissure of Sylvius (Fig. 17), then guiding structures for the spread of the perifocal edema are lacking. In the periventricular white matter of the left anterior horn, the density is decreased. We do not consider this zone of decreased density in the periventricular tissue as edema distant from the tumor, but as an expression of transependymal transfer of fluid into the white matter by a partial hydrocephalus under pressure [21, 43, 77].

Oligodendrogliomas II without calcification cannot be differentiated from astrocytomas II in the computed tomogram. Likewise, it is not possible to differentiate tumor tis-

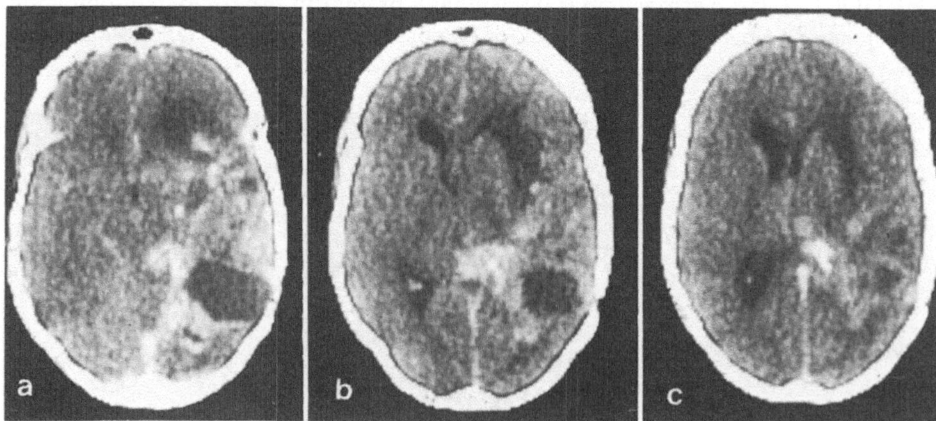

Fig. 18 a–c. Oligodendroglioma (recurred) in the right-temporo-occipital area. Spread of edema is only possible along the white matter between the Sylvian fissure and the adjacent basal ganglia. The internal capsule is enlarged (**b, c**). The edema reaches the frontal aspect of the lateral ventricle, but extends no further drainage of edema into ventricle

sue and perifocal edema. *Anaplastic and polymorphic oligodendrogliomas,* in contrast and independent of the type of tumor show obvious perifocal edema in the adjacent white matter (Fig. 18) in the computed tomogram.

Gliobastomas, in accordance with their "multiform structure", appear in the plain CT with mixed zones, i.e. hypodense, isodense and hyperdense zones. Generally speaking, a demarcation of the tumor tissue from the surrounding edema is not possible in the plain CT, since hypodense areas of the tumor and edematous cerebral tissue have identical absorption values. After giving contrast medium, the glioblastomas are seen in the computed tomogram in their true extent, and demarcation from perifocal edema is then possible (Fig. 13). Incipient glioblastomas (12% of our investigated series) appear as areas of decreased density without appreciable take-up of contrast medium; differentiation of tumor tissue and edema is not possible.

Pilocytic astrocytomas (formerly known as cerebellar astrocytomas, cerebellar spongioblastomas, polar spongioblastomas, optic nerve gliomas, hypothalamus gliomas, juvenile astrocytomas and infundibulomas) occur mainly in children and adolescents. We present some of the numerous appearances of pilocytic astrocytomas in the computed tomogram which are of importance for the diagnosis or differential diagnosis of brain edema. Pilocytic astrocytomas in the pons are characterized in the plain CT by low absorption values, and frequently take up contrast medium in a patchy fashion (Fig. 19). Parts of the tumor cannot be differentiated from any edema which may be present.

In some cases, pilocytic astrocytomas of the cerebral hemispheres appear very similar to the cystic pilocytic astrocytomas of the posterior cranial fossa in the computed tomogram. In the plain CT, more or less extensive circular zones of decreased density are present, and their absorption values also resemble those of brain edema. Their smooth boundary and the lack of configurative reference to the centrum ovale exclude any confusion with edema. After administration of contrast medium, the relatively small solid parts of the tumor appear as nodular regions of increased density (Fig. 20).

The difference between the shapeless appearance of the tumor cysts or the almost filigree pattern of the cerebral white matter is particularly clear in Fig. 20 b.

Plexus papillomas, which occur in the trigonal region of the lateral ventricle, show zones of decreased density in the adjacent white matter. The absorption values of these zones of decreased density correspond to those of perifocal brain edema, but it is possible that there has been a transependymal transfer of fluid from the ventricle

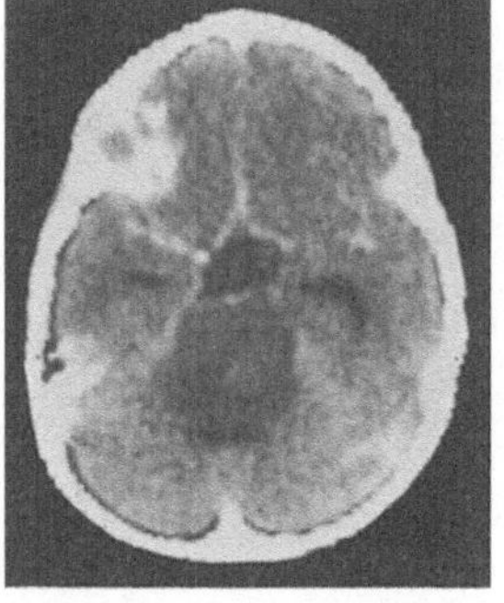

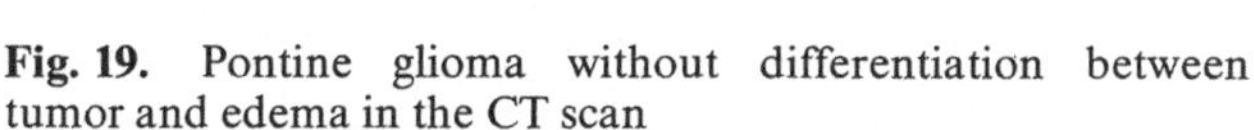

Fig. 19. Pontine glioma without differentiation between tumor and edema in the CT scan

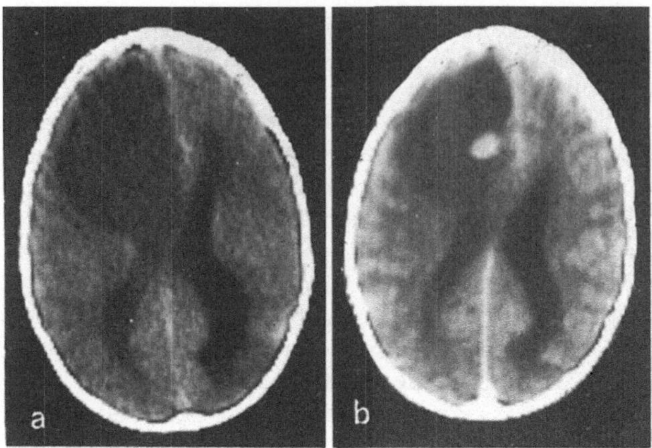

Fig. 20 a, b. Pilocytic astrocytoma in the left cerebral hemisphere. Enhancement at the edge of the tumor without any edema in the neighbouring white matter

enlarged by the tumor. Differentiation based on the absorption values is not possible. Since, however, these zones of decreased density can only be detected where a congested residue of fluid is visible on the surface of the tumor, it is more probable that passive transport of the fluid under pressure into the adjacent white matter has occurred through the ependyma of the ventricular wall, which has altered permeability.

Meningiomas with a figure of 16%, are the second largest group of tumors in our series. Within the large group of meningiomas, we found very large differences in respect of the frequency and extent of perifocal edema (Table 8). On the one hand,

Table 8. Perifocal edema in menigiomas ($n = 267$)

Site	No. of tumors	Edema
Clivus	2	0
Suprasellar region	14	0
Ventricle	2	1
Cerebellopontine angle	24	2 (8%)
Tentorium	20	2 (10%)
Temporobasal region	18	2 (11%)
Convexity	84	60 (71%)
occipital	8	4 (50%)
parietal	32	19 (61%)
frontal	34	27 (79%)
temporal	10	10 (100%)
Spenoidal wing	44	25 (57%)
lateral	18	6 (33%)
medial	26	19 (73%)
Falx	30	20 (67%)
Dura-falx angle parasagittal	20	18 (90%)
Frontobasal region	18	18 (100%)

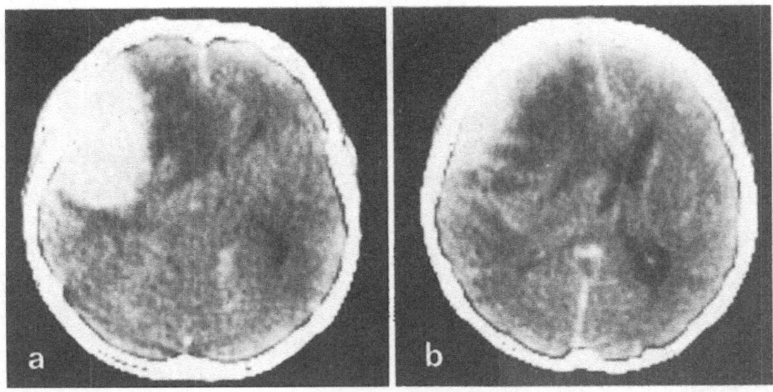

Fig. 21 a, b. Convexity meningioma on the left side with finely pointed surface and perifocal edema grade II

the variable location of the meningiomas is very important for the presence or absence of perifocal edema, since this, with some exceptions, spreads exclusively in the white matter. Suprasellar meningiomas and clivus meningiomas had no contact with the white matter, so the prerequisite for the detection of any edema by computed tomography was lacking. Intraventricular meningiomas, which also lack contact with the white matter, have a special position and they present the same problems as the plexus papillomas.

We observed in a number of the cases of convexity meningiomas irregular, in some cases pointed boundaries on the surface of the tumor against the brain tissue (Figs. 21 a, b). These meningiomas always appeared in the computed tomogram with perifocal brain edema, in contrast to the smooth boundaries of the convexity meningiomas which only very rarely showed perifocal edema. During operation we found in meningiomas, with irregular boundaries in the CT, that the almost mirror-like fine tumor capsule was absent where the nodular tumor contours were present in the computed tomogram. Meningioma tissue in these regions lay "bare" in the adjacent, mainly edematous, brain tissue.

The loss of the "tumor capsule" and the atrophy of the pia mater, by which a meningioma is demarcated from the brain tissue, are in our opinion important morphological prerequisites for the extension of brain edema, detectable by computed tomography, in convexity meningiomas. During operation we also observed in large convexity meningiomas that the peritumoral brain tissue was altered in color and was necrotic in consistency. The expanding meningioma likewise makes contact with the white matter of the cerebrum via the ischemic necrosis of this zone of the cerebral cortex displaced by the tumor [46]. Extremely large meningiomas show no perifocal edema if they impinge on the boundary of the cerebral lobe or are bounded by masses of grey matter or by cisterns (Fig. 22). Central frontobasel meningiomas typically show bilateral edema in both frontal lobes (Fig. 14); however, if frontobasal meningiomas develop more or less unilaterally, they are then also accompanied by unilaterally predominating but bilateral edema (Fig. 23).

The meningiomas investigated and operated on by us were histologically classified as arachnothelial, fibroblastic and arachnothelial-fibroblastic tumors. For each of

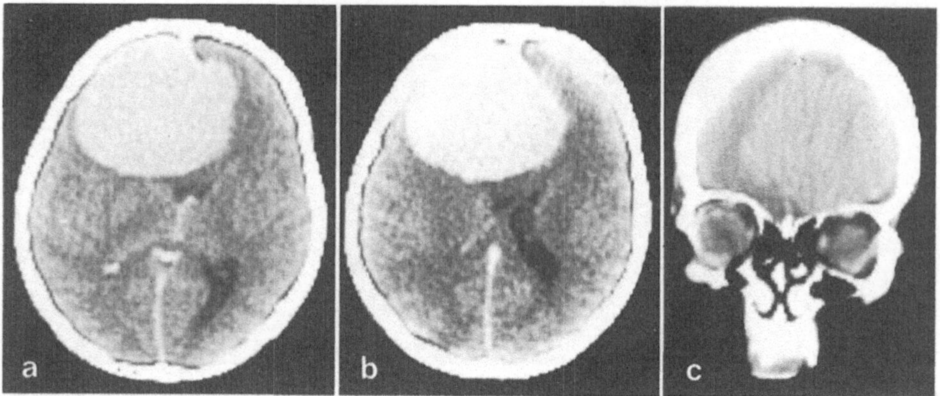

Fig. 22a–c. Huge falx meningioma extending to opposite side. Sharp limitation by the Sylvian fissure and both lateral ventricles (**a**). Slight edema in the white matter of the adjacent frontal lobe

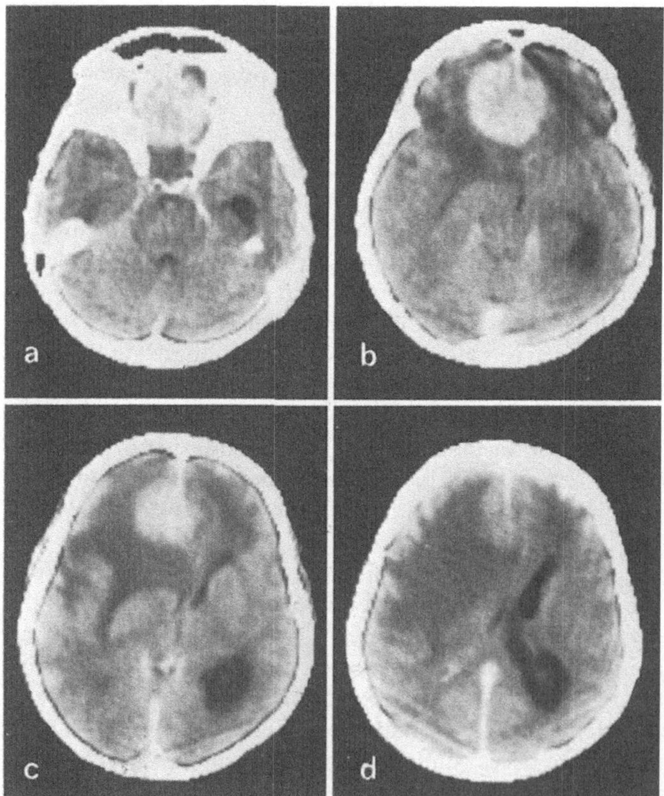

Fig. 23a–d. Olfactory groove meningioma, more on the left side, with marked edema in the white matter on the left

these three types of meningioma, there is a variant with an increased tendency to grow. If comparison is made of the frequency of edema in these six histologically differentiated meningiomas, then it emerges that the fibroblastic meningiomas have the lowest frequency of edema (43%). The arachnothelial meningiomas show an equal incidence of edema as the arachnothelial-fibroblastic meningiomas (50–52%). However, the frequency of edema rises by 30–50% in fibroblastic or arachnothelial-fibroblastic meningiomas with increased tendency to grow. Vassilouthis and Ambrose [83] found similar results.

The 575 *brain metastases* are the third largest group of tumors in our series, with a proportion of 15.3%, lying next to the glioblastomas (18.9%) and the meningiomas (16.1%). The most frequent were bronchial carcinoma metastases with a proportion of 33.4%, followed by metastases from carcinoma of the breast (18.5%), metastases from malignant melanomas (10%), from renal carcinoma (6.5%), from carcinomas of the gastro-intestinal tract (7.7%) and a group of metastases from carcinomas of very differing origins (26.9%). Of the metastases in our patients 87% were surrounded by perifocal brain edema. There are many reports that brain metastases frequently show perifocal brain edema in the computed tomogram [8, 12, 18, 51, 64], however, no percentage frequency has yet been indicated. Computed tomograms give the impression that isolated brain metastases have more extensive edema than glioblastomas or meningiomas (Fig. 8). The "discrepancy" between the size of a metastasis and the spread of the perifocal edema results from the fact that the metastases are on average smaller than glioblastomas. Thus the smaller metastases, which themselves require less space from the adjacent white matter, have relatively more space available for the expansion of the perifocal edema.

Brain metastases are, next to glioblastomas, the only tumors in our series in which we observed spreading of the perifocal edema also into the grey matter structures. Multiple metastases produce multiple areas of perifocal edema.

Perifocal Edema with Expanding Intracranial Lesions not Caused by Tumors

After completion of the phlegmonous phase, *brain abscesses* of various origins appear in the computed tomogram as localized expanding lesions. In the plain CT, the abscess, surrounded by a large zone of decreased density, is not generally visible. This extended zone of decreased density represents not only the abscess with a more or less developed wall of granulation but also the perifocal edema. Occasionally, within this large zone of decreased density, a discrete ring structure can be seen (Fig. 24). After administration of contrast medium, the density in the ring-like granulation wall (abscess capsule) significantly increases, so that the oval or circular, usually smoothly circumscribed abscess, can be unambiguously demarcated from the perifocal edema [3, 32, 50, 55, 73]. This typical computed tomographic appearance of a smoothly circumscribed ring structure round a zone of decreased density and within a irregularly outlined zone of decreased density (perifocal edema) can produce, in isolated cases, difficulties in the differential diagnosis, and can be impossible to differentiate from a central necrotic glioblastoma, a metastasis or a tumor resection cavity in the early postoperative phase [34]. The perifocal edema of brain abscesses does not differ from perifocal brain tumor edema either in the pattern of spread or in the absorption values.

The 52 brain abscesses diagnosed in our clinic by computed tomography and confirmed by operation, were surrounded by perifocal brain edema in 88.5% of the cases. Of the 46 patients with a brain abscess, nine (19.6%) showed perifocal edema degree I, 33 patients (71.8%) were found to have an edema degree II and four patients (8.6%) showed an edema degree III in the computed tomogram. Reports by New et al. [54], Nielsen and Gyldensted [57] and Stevens et al. [78] show that brain abscesses are surrounded by perifocal edema in more than 80% of the cases. However, based on our investigations, we must state that the frequency and spread of the

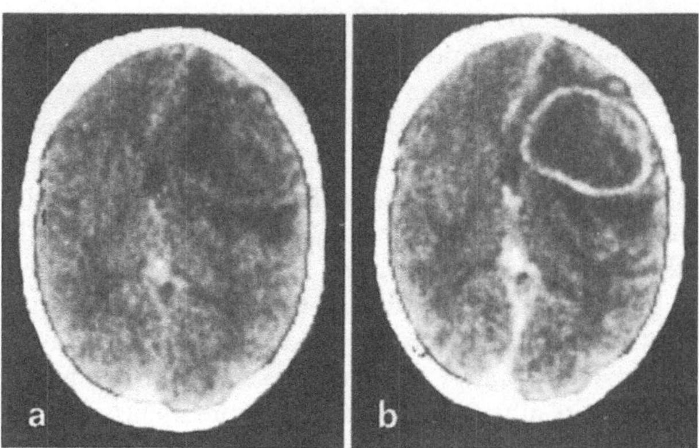

Fig. 24 a, b. Abscess, right frontal region. After administration of contrast medium enhancement of the capsule with slight perifocal edema

perifocal edema does not represent a differential diagnostic criterion for a brain abscess, since both glioblastomas with an edema incidence of 92% and brain metastases with an edema incidence of 87% are approximately equally frequently surrounded by perifocal edema as are brain abscesses and, in cases of doubt, cannot be differentiated from them in the computed tomogram.

Massive intracerebral bleeding of various origins appears in the acute stage as sharply localized zones of increased density in the computed tomogram. The observation which we reported in an earlier publication [22] that 577 patients with spontaneous intracerebral bleeding in the acute phase investigated by computed tomography showed no detectable brain edema, can now be made more precise on the basis of further investigations. In control investigations using computed tomography on 90 patients with massive spontaneous intracerebral bleeding, of which one half were conservatively treated, we observed in the computed tomogram at the earliest after 24 hours a perifocal edema in the cerebral white matter adjacent to the bleeding. The frequency of the perifocal edema (50%) of this series of investigations corresponds to the frequency of edema which we found in the patients in the combined study published in 1979, and which was reported by Clasen et al. [14]. Within the first 12–24 hours, however, the computed tomographic image, apart from the occurrence of perifocal edema, changes as a result of absorptive processes in the boundary region between hematoma and adjacent brain tissue. In this early phase, we have observed a narrow limbus of decreased density in the periphery of the hematoma (Fig. 25). This limbus is regarded as a zone of absorption [14, 23, 31]. In the literature up to now, the morphological correlative for this so-called absorption zone has been assumed to be absorptive processes in the periphery of the hematoma. In 18 of 90 cases, we established that the diameter of the hematoma in the computed tomogram did not alter in the first 24–48 hours after the appearance of the so-called absorption zone. The limbus of decreased density around the large hematoma which is unaltered in the computed tomogram, may thus correspond to a process in the adjacent brain tissue leading to a change in density. This is either the early phase of a perifocally expanding edema or the computed tomographic appearance

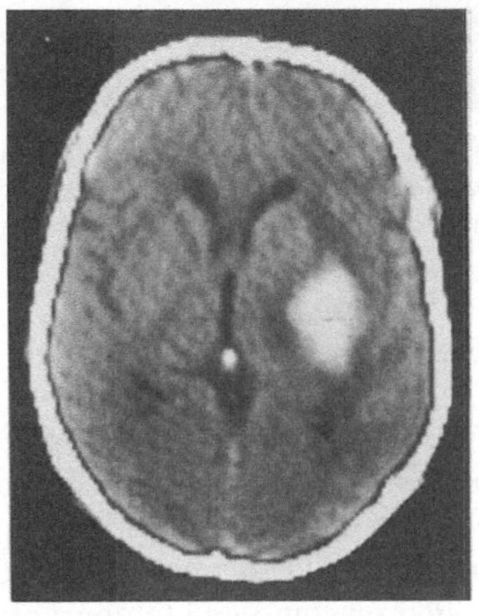

Fig. 25. Basal ganglia hemorrhage on the right side, three days old. The area of low density spreads into the external capsule and behind the Sylvian fissure

associated with the clearing of the raggedly disintegrated brain tissue of the wall of the hematoma cavity by fat granular cells [24]. After 3–4 days, the limbus of decreased density becomes larger with simultaneous decrease in the diameter of the hematoma. In this phase, three alterations can be detected in the computed tomogram:

1. The hematoma appears with a smaller diameter in the unenhanced image.
2. The hematoma is surrounded by a more or less extensive zone of decreased density, which extends into the adjacent white matter (Fig. 25).
3. After administration of contrast medium, a narrow ring of increased density appears concentrically round the hematoma; between this ring and the hematoma, an equally narrow limbus of decreased density is visible (Fig. 26).

These CT findings, based on the pathological-anatomical investigations, may, in our opinion, be interpreted as follows:

1. In recent massive intracerebral bleeding, it cannot be decided in the plain computed tomogram whether the limbus of decreased density corresponds to the early stage of perifocal brain edema or absorptive processes in the surroundings of the hematoma.
2. Only after giving contrast medium can the absorption zones in the periphery of the hematoma be differentiated from the glio-fibrillary limbus formed around the cavity of the hematoma (contrast-intensified ring) and the perifocal edema.

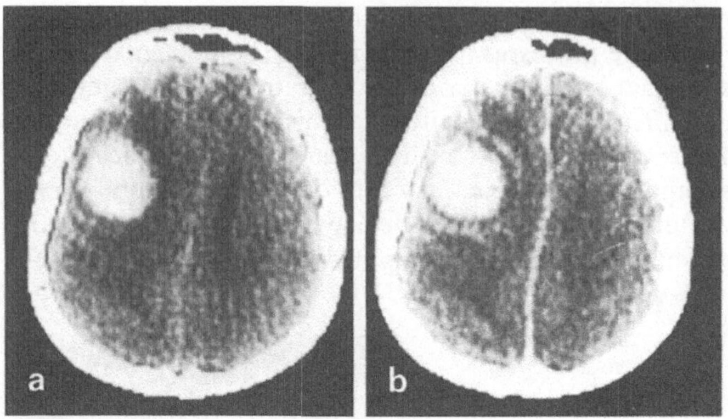

Fig. 26 a, b. Intracerebral hemorrhage four days old. Close to the hemorrhage an unclear zone with reduced density (**a**). After administration of contrast medium ringshape enhancement with distinction between hematoma and edema

Edema in Cerebral Infarction

The brain edema described up to now and detectable by computed tomography in intrinsic brain tumors, meningiomas, metastases, abscesses and spontaneous intracerebral bleeding correspond to vasogenic brain edema as defined by Klatzo (1967). In contrast to this perifocal edema, which appears almost exclusively in the white matter on computed tomography (for exceptions, see under glioblastomas and brain metastases), edema can be detected in cerebral arterial vascular occlusions, both in the white and in the grey matter. After an arterial vascular occlusion, a cerebral vein thrombosis or an occlusion of a large sinus, the entire vascular circulation area appears as a homogeneous dark zone with decreased absorption of radiation. These changes in density, according to our observations however, are not immediately detectable, but appear at the earliest four and a half hours after the acute episode and can then be clearly depicted after electronic image manipulation (narrowing the window width). Aulich and Fenske [4] report that three hours is the minimum for the development of ischemic alterations detectable by computed tomography. Four hours after the acute event, they observed changes in density in the computed tomogram in 5% of all acute cerebral ischemias. After eight hours 19% of the patients and after 24 hours 44% of the patients showed ischemic alterations in the computed tomogram. Signs of a brain infarction are detectable by computed tomography in 75% of the patients after 48 hours. Areas of infarction in the computed tomogram were seen in 95% of the patients after a week. We were able to confirm these time-dependent alterations in the computed tomogram in our investigations (Fig. 27).
Bartko et al. [6] and Shaw et al. [75] describe brain edema in the initial phase of stroke as a cytotoxic edema. The ischemia leads primarily to a disturbance of cell metabolism with consecutive cellular hydrops and not to a change in the permeability of the blood-brain barrier with extravascular fluid accumulation. This vasogenic edema can first appear 5–6 hours after the vascular occlusion and reaches its maximum after 1–2 days [10, 58]. Assuming that the results of these animal experiments are also true for the pathology of infarction edema in humans, then the

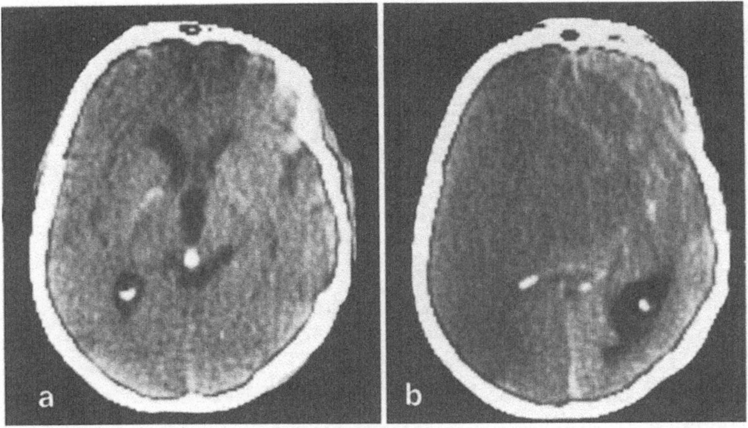

Fig. 27. a Slight edema on first day and **b** extensive edema due to infarction of the left hemisphere, two days after occlusion of the internal carotid artery

findings in the computed tomogram are explicable. The detection of the cytotoxic edema in initial phase when there is only slight intracellular take-up of water is not possible with the density resolving power of the scanning equipment available at present. Changes in density in the CT appear only after secondary formation and expansion of the vasogenic brain edema with a substantially larger increase in the water content in the white matter. Torack et al. [79, 80] have detected in autopsy material that the water content in brain infarction increases in the grey matter from 83.35% to 85.56% and in the white matter from 70.95% to 80.85%. These results also confirm that the changes which are relevant for the changes in density visible in the computed tomogram, occur mostly in the white matter. Shaw et al. [75] and Ng et al. [56] have already referred to this dilation reaction of the white matter on cerebral infarction in humans. In extensive infarcts after occlusion of the internal carotid artery or the middle cerebral artery, the X-ray absorption values are decreased not only in the white matter affected but also in the grey matter of the basal ganglia and of the cortex (Fig. 27). These edema-dependent decreases in density in the grey matter, which are only extremely rarely observed in perifocal edema, can be explained by the fact that the decreased tissue perfusion caused by an increase in volume (as a result of the expanding secondary vasogenic edema) increases the primary ischemic effect on the grey matter and leads to an increased up-take of water [27]. The average decrease in density in recent ischemic infarcts is 20–30 Hounsfield units. Both the absorption values as well as the outlines of a recent brain infarct change subsequently. The area affected by infarct edema becomes smaller and the initially diffuse demarcation from the unaffected brain tissue becomes sharper in outline. The absorption values decrease continuously in large brain infarcts until, after 6–8 weeks, they correspond to fluid density values [33, 40].

We have not yet been able to clarify by tissue analysis whether these low density values in the circumscribed parenchymatous defects can be attributed exclusively to the presence of fluid. It cannot be ruled out that fat-containing substances in these scarred regions exert an influence on the decrease in density. In less extensive par-

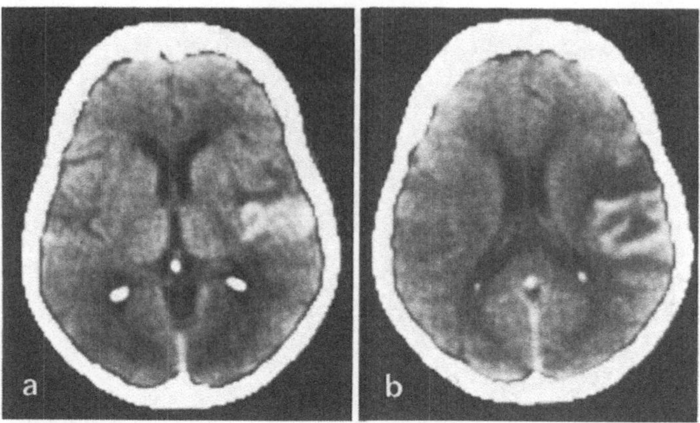

Fig. 28 a, b. Regional infarction of the territory of the middle cerebral artery. Enhancement inside the territory, with luxury perfusion 20 days after onset of stroke. The picture resembles a cortical glioma

tial infarcts, the density values can subsequently become normal so that the computed tomographic image appears quite unremarkable.

In the course of brain infarct control investigations both the disturbance of the blood-brain barrier and also the luxury perfusion can be detected by computed tomography. Intravenous administration of contrast medium leads either to ring-like structures as a result of a contrast enhancement in the periphery of the infarct or to cord-like or to garland-like images as the result of an increase in contrast in the region of the cortex (Fig. 28). These computed tomographic images can only lead to confusion with neoplastic lesions when the history and clinical findings are ignored when assessing the computed tomograms. Homogeneous contrast intensification arises both in primary hypodense as well as in isodense infarction areas. These phenomena detectable by computed tomography can usually no longer be detected from the 4th to 5th week onwards.

References

1. Ambrose J (1973) Computerized transverse axial scanning (tomography). Part II, Clinical application. Brit J Radiol 46, 1023–1047
2. Arimitsu T, Di Chiro G, Brooks RA, Smith PB (1977) White – grey matter differentiation in computed tomography. J Comp Assist Tomogr 1, 437–442
3. Aulich A, Lange S, Steinhoff H, Schindler E, Wende S (1976) Diagnosis and follow-up studies in brain abscesses using CT. In: Cranial computerized tomography. Lanksch W, Kazner E (eds). Springer, Berlin Heidelberg New York, pp 366–371
4. Aulich A, Fenske A (1977) Das Computertomogramm des Schlaganfalles. Akt Neurol 4, 129–140
5. Baker HL, Campbell JK, Houser OW, Reese DF, Sheedy PF, Holman CB, Kurland RL (1974) Computer assisted tomography of the head. An early evaluation. Mayo Clinic Proceedings 49, 17–27
6. Bartko D, Reulen HJ, Koch H, Schürmann K (1972) Effect of dexamethasone on the early edema following occlusion of the middle cerebral artery in cats. In: Steroids and brain edema. Reulen HJ, Schürmann K (eds). Springer, Berlin Heidelberg New York, pp 127–137

7. Ben-Shmuel A (1964) Elektronenmikroskopische Untersuchungen über das im Marklager lokalisierte Hirnödem. Z Zellforsch 64, 523–532
8. Black P (1979) Brain metastases: current status and recommended guidelines for management. Neurosurgery 5, 617–631
9. Blakemore WF (1969) The fate of escaped plasma protein after thermal necrosis of the rat brain; an electron microscope study. J Neuropath exp Neurol 28, 139–152
10. O'Brien MD, Jordan MM, Waltz AG (1974) Ischemic cerebral edema and the blood-brain barrier. Distributions of pertechnetate, albumin, sodium and antipyrine in brains of cats after occlusion of the middle cerebral artery. Arch Neurol 30, 461–465
11. Brooks RA, Di Chiro G, Keller MR (1980) Explanation of cerebral white – grey contrast in computed tomography. J Comp Assist Tomogr 4, 489–491
12. Chiras J, Gueye M, Salomon G (1978) The role of computerised tomography in the diagnosis of cerebral metastases. J Neuroradiology 5, 333–349
13. Cho ZH, Tsai CM, Wilson G (1975) Study of contrast and modulation mechanisms in x-ray/photon transverse axial transmission tomography. Phys Med Biol 20, 879–889
14. Clasen RA, Huckman MS, Pandolfy S, Laing I, Jacobs J (1976) Computed tomography of vasogenic cerebral edema. In: Dynamics of brain edema. Pappius HM, Feindel W (eds). Springer, Berlin Heidelberg New York, pp 278–282
15. David E, Marx I, David H (1967) Zur Feinstruktur des experimentell erzeugten subakuten und chronischen Hirnödems. Acta Neuropathologica 9, 217–232
16. Davis OD, Pressman BD (1974) Computerized tomography of the brain. Radiol Clin North America XII 2, 297–313
17. Dubal L, Wiggli U (1977) Tomochemistry of the brain. J Comp Assist Tomogr 1, 300–307
18. Elke M, Hünig R, Wiggli U, Fridrich R, Müller HR, Wüthrich R (1976) The diagnosis of intracranial metastases: the efficiency of CT and scintigraphy in patients investigated by both methods. In: Cranial computerized tomography. Lanksch W, Kazner E (eds). Springer, Berlin Heidelberg New York, pp 171–176
19. Fenske A, Samii M, Reulen HJ, Hey O (1973) Extracellular space and electrolyte distribution in cortex and white matter of dog brain in cold induced oedema. Acta Neurochir 28, 81–94
20. Fischgold H (1973) L'EMI-Scanner. J Radiol Electrol Med Nucl 54, 1–5
21. Greitz T, Hindmarsh T (1974) Computer assisted tomography of intracranial CSF circulation using a water-soluble contrast medium. Acta radiol Diagnosis 15, 497
22. Grumme Th, Lanksch W, Kretzschmar K (1979) Intrakranielle Blutungen im Computertomogramm. Dtsch Ärzteblatt 24, 1627–1634
23. Grumme Th, Lanksch W, Wende S (1976) Diagnosis of spontaneous intracerebral hemorrhaged by computerized tomography. In: Cranial computerized tomography. Lanksch W, Kazner E (eds). Springer, Berlin Heidelberg New York, pp 284–290
24. Hamperl H (1960) Lehrbuch der Allgemeinen Pathologie und der Pathologischen Anatomie. 24./25. Aufl, Springer, Berlin Göttingen Heidelberg, pp 424–426
25. Herrmann HD, Neuenfeldt D (1972) Development and regression of a disturbance of the blood-brain-barrier and of edema in tissue surrounding a circumscribed cold lesion. Exp Neurol 34, 115–120
26. Hochwald GM, Marlin AE, Wald A, Malhan C (1976) Movement of water between blood, brain and CSF in cerebral edema. In: Dynamics of brain edema, Pappius HM, Feindel W (eds). Springer, Berlin Heidelberg New York, pp 129–137
27. Hossmann KA, Schuier FJ (1979) Pathophysiology of stroke edema. In: Brain and heart infarct II, Zülch KJ, Kaufmann W, Hossmann KA, Hossmann V (eds). Springer, Berlin Heidelberg New York, pp 119–129
28. Hossmann KA, Wilmes F, Blöink M (1979) Experimental peritumorous edema of the cat brain. 1st. International Ernst Reuter Symposium. Brain edema
29. Hounsfield GN (1973) Computerized transverse axial scanning (tomography): Part I. Description of system. Brit J Radiol 46, 1016–1022
30. Huber P (1979) Zerebrale Angiographie für Klinik und Praxis. Krayenbühl H, Yazargil MG (eds). Thieme, Stuttgart, pp 244–256

31. Huk W, Schiefer W (1976) Computerized tomography (Siretom) of acute cerebrovascular events. In: Cranial computerized tomography. Lanksch W, Kazner E (eds). Springer, Berlin Heidelberg New York, pp 264–272
32. Joubert MJ, Stephanou S (1977) Computerized tomography and surgical treatment in intracranial suppuration. J Neurosurg 47, 73–78
33. Kazner E, Lanksch W, Steinhoff H, Wilske J (1975) Die axiale Computer-Tomographie des Gehirnschädels. Fortschr Neurol Psychiat 43, 487–574
34. Kazner E, Wende S, Grumme Th, Lanksch W, Stochdorph O (1981) Computertomographie intrakranieller Tumoren aus klinischer Sicht. Springer, Berlin Heidelberg New York
35. Klatzo I, Piraux A, Laskowski EJ (1958) The relationship between edema, blood-brain barrier and tissue elements in local brain injury. J Neuropath exp Neurol 17, 548–564
36. Klatzo I, Wisniewski H, Steinwall O, Streicher E (1967) Dynamics of cold injury edema. In: Brain edema. Klatzo I, Seitelberger F (eds). Springer, Berlin Heidelberg New York, pp 554–563
37. Kodoma JK, Butler WM, Tusing TW (1973) Jodothalamate: a new intravascular radiopaque medium with unusual pharmacotoxic inertness. Experimental and Molecular Pathology, Supplement II: 65–80
38. Ladurner G (1978) Die Bestimmung des zerebralen Blutvolumens mit der Computertomographie in grauer und weißer Substanz. Fortschr Neurol Psychiatr 46, 369–381
39. Lalli AF (1980) Contrast media reactions: data analysis and hypothesis. Radiology 134, 1–12
40. Lanksch W, Oettinger W, Baethmann A, Kazner E (1976) CT findings in brain edema compared with direct chemical analysis of tissue samples. In: Dynamics of Brain Edema. Pappius HM, Feindel W (eds). Springer, Berlin Heidelberg New York, pp 283–287
41. Lanksch W, Kazner E (1976) CT findings in brain edema. In: Cranial computerized tomography. Lanksch W, Kazner E (eds). Springer, Berlin Heidelberg New York, pp 344–355
42. Lanksch W, Oettinger W, Baethmann A (1977) Diagnosis of brain edema using CT. In: Computer assisted tomography. Kühler WJ (ed). Excerpta Medica, Amsterdam Oxford, pp 13–25
43. Lanksch W, Grumme Th, Kazner E, Baethmann A CT evaluation of peritumoral brain edema (in press). 1st. International Ernst-Reuter-Symposium. Brain edema. 12.–15. Sept. 1979, Berlin
44. Lanksch W, Ringel K (1981) Zur Diagnostik und Therapie von zerebralen Nieren-Karzinom-Metastasen. In: Diagnostik und Therapie des Nierenkarzinoms. Schmiedt E, Bauer H-W (eds). Zuckschwerdt, München, pp 160–165
45. Lanksch W (1981) Computertomographie intrakranieller Tumoren aus klinischer Sicht. Kazner E, Wende S, Grumme Th, Lanksch W, Stochdorph O (eds). Springer, Berlin Heidelberg New York
46. Lanksch W (1981) Grundlagen zur Diagnose des Hirnödems im Computertomogramm. Computertomographische und biochemische Untersuchungsergebnisse von Ödemen bei Hirntumoren, Hirnabszessen und zerebralen Gefäßprozessen. Habilitationsschrift, München
47. Meinig G, Aulich A, Wende S, Reulen HJ (1976) The effect of dexamethasone and diuretics on peritumoral brain edema: cooperative study of tissue water content and CT. In: Dynamics of brain edema. Pappius HM, Feindel W (eds). Springer, Berlin Heidelberg New York, pp 301–305
48. Meinig G, Reulen HJ, Schürmann K Clinical, chemical and CT-evaluation of short-time and long-time edema-therapy with dexamethasone and diuretics (in press). 1st. International Ernst Reuter Symposium. Brain edema. 12.–15. Sept. 1979, Berlin
49. Melartin E, Tuohimaa PJ, Dabb R (1970) Neurotoxicity of iothalamates and diatrizoates. I. Significance of concentration and cation. Invest Radiol 5, 13–21
50. Moseley IF, Claveria LE, du Boulay GH (1977) The role of C.A.T. in the diagnosis and management of intracranial infections. In: Computerised axial tomography in clinical practice, du Boulay GH, Moseley IF (eds). Springer, Berlin Heidelberg New York, pp 182–190

51. Nadjmi M, Piepgras U, Vogelsang H (1981) Kranielle Computertomographie. Thieme, Stuttgart New York, pp 324–335
52. New PFJ, Scott WR, Schnur JA, Davies KR, Taveras JM, Hochberg FH (1975) Computed tomography with the EMI scanner in the diagnosis of primary and metastatic intracranial neoplasms. Radiology 114, 75–87
53. New PFJ, Scott WR (1975) Computed tomography of the brain and orbit (EMI scanning). Williams and Wilkins, Baltimore, pp 263–267
54. New PFJ, Davies KR, Ballantine HT (1976) Computed tomography in cerebral abscess. Radiology 121, 641–646
55. Newton TH, Norman D, Alvord Ellsworth C, Shaw Ch (1977) The CT scan in infections diseases of the CNS. In: Computed tomography. Norman D, Korobkin M, Newton TH (eds). Mosby, St. Louis, pp 317–338
56. Ng LKY, Nimmammitya J (1970) Massive cerebral infarction with severe brain swelling. Stroke 1, 158–163
57. Nielsen H, Gyldensted C (1977) Computed tomography in the diagnosis of cerebral abscess. Neuroradiology 12, 207–217
58. Olsson Y, Crowell RM, Klatzo I (1971) The blood-brain barrier to protein tracers in focal cerebral ischemia and infarction caused by occlusion of the middle cerebral artery. Acta Neuropathol 18, 89–102
59. Ommaya AK (1973) Computerized axial tomography of the head: The EMI-Scanner, a new device for direct examination of the brain "in vivo". Surg Neurol q, 217–222
60. Pappius HM, Gulati DR (1963) Water and electrolyte content of cerebral tissues in experimentally induced edema. Acta Neuropath 2, 451–460
61. Paxton R, Amrose J (1974) The EMI scanner. A brief review of the first 650 patients. Brit J Radiol 47, 530–564
62. Perry BJ, Bridges C (1973) Computerized transverse axial scanning (tomography): Part 3. Radiation dose considerations. Brit J Radiol 46, 1048–1051
63. Phelps ME, Hoffmann EJ, Ter-Pogossian MM (1975) Attenuation coefficients of various body tissues, fluids, and lesions at photon energies of 18 to 136 KeV. Radiology 117, 573–583
64. Potts DG, Abbot GF, v. Sneidern JV (1980) National cancer institute study: Evaluation of computed tomography in the diagnosis of intracranial neoplasms. III. Metastatic tumors. Radiology 136, 657–664
65. Reulen HJ Dynamics of resolution of vasogenic edema (in press). 1st. International Ernst Reuter Symposium. Brain Edema. 12.–15. Sept. 1979, Berlin
66. Reulen HJ, Graham A, Fenske A, Tsuyumu M, Klatzo I (1976) The role of tissue pressure and bulk flow in the formation and resolution of cold-induced edema. In: Dynamics of brain edema. Pappius HM, Feindel W (eds). Springer, Berlin Heidelberg New York, pp 103–112
67. Reulen HJ, Graham R, Klatzo I (1975) Development of pressure gradients within brain tissue during the formation of vasogenic brain edema. In: Intracranial pressure II. Lundberg N, Ponten U, Brock M (eds). Springer, Berlin Heidelberg New York, pp 233–238
68. Reulen HJ, Graham A, Spatz M, Klatzo I (1977) Role of pressure gradients and bulk flow in dynamics of vasogenic brain edema. J Neurosurg 46, 24–35
69. Reulen HJ, Hadjidimos A, Schürmann K (1972) The effect of dexamethasone on water and electrolyte content and on CBF in perifocal brain edema in man. In: Steroids and Brain Edema. Reulen HJ, Schürmann K (eds). Springer, Berlin Heidelberg New York, pp 239–252
70. Reulen HJ, Kreysch HG (1973) Measurement of brain tissue pressure in cold-induced cerebral edema. Acta Neurochir 29, 29–40
71. Reulen HJ, Medzihradsky F, Enzenbach R, Marguth F, Brendel W (1969) Electrolytes, fluids and energy metabolism in cerebral edema in man. Arch Neurol 21, 517–525
72. Rieth KG, Fujiwara K, Di Chiro G, Klatzo I, Brooks R, Johnston GS, O'Connor ChM, Mitchell LG (1980) Serial measurements of CT attenuation and specific gravity in experimental cerebral edema. Radiology 135, 343–348
73. Schiefer W, Huk W (1976) Computerized tomographic findings with brain abscesses. In: Cranial Computerized Tomography. Lanksch W, Kazner E (eds). Springer, Berlin Heidelberg New York, pp 360–365

74. Schmiedek P, Baethmann A, Schneider E, Oettinger W, Enzenbach R, Marguth F, Brendel W (1972) The effect of aldosterone and aldosterone-antagonist on the metabolism of perifocal brain edema in man. In: Steroids and brain edema. Reulen HJ, Schürmann K (eds). Springer, Berlin Heidelberg New York, pp 203–210
75. Shaw CM, Alvord EC, Berry RG (1959) Swelling of the brain following ischemic infarction with arterial occlusion. Arch Neurol 1, 161–177
76. Speck U, Nagel R, Leistenschneider W, Mützel W (1977) Pharmakokinetik und Biotransformation neuer Röntgenkontrastmittel für die Uro- und Angiographie beim Patienten. Fortschr Röntgenstr 127, 270–274
77. Sprung Ch, Grumme Th (1979) Use of CT cisternography, RISA cisternography, and the infusion test for predicting shunting results in normal pressure hydrocephalus. (NPH). Advances in Neurosurgery, vol 7. Springer, Berlin Heidelberg New York, pp 350–360
78. Stevens EA, Norman D, Kramer RA, Messina AB, Newton TH (1978) Computed tomography brain scanning in intraparenchymal pyogenic abscesses. Amer J Roentgenol 130, 111–114
79. Torack RM, Alcala H, Gado M (1976) Water, specific gravity and histology as determinants of diagnostic computerized tomography (CCT). In: Dynamic of brain edema. Pappius HM, Feindel W (eds). Springer, Berlin Heidelberg New York, pp 271–277
80. Torack RM, Alcala H, Gado M, Burton R (1976) Correlative assay of computerized cranial tomography, water content and specific gravity in normal and pathological postmortem brain. J Neuropath exp Neurol 35, 385–392
81. Torack RM, Terry RD, Zimmermann HM (1960) The fine structure of cerebral fluid accumulation. II. Swelling produced by triethyl tin poisoning and its comparison with that in the human brain. Amer J Pathol 36, 237–287
82. Tuohimaa PJ, Melartin E (1970) Neurotoxicity of iothalamates and diatrizoates. II. Historadioautographic study of rat brains with 131-iodine-tagged contrast media. Invest Radiol 5, 22–29
83. Vassilouthis J, Ambrose J (1979) Computerized tomography scanning appearances of intracranial meningomas. – An attempt to predict the histological features – Brain edema. J Neurosurg 50, 320–327
84. WHO-Klassifikation (1979) Histological typing of tumours of the central nervous system. Internat Histol Classific of Tumours No. 21 (Zülch, KJ, ed.), World Health Organisation, Geneva
85. Willis RA (1948) Pathology of tumours. Butterworth & Co., London
86. Yates AJ, Thelmo W, Pappius HM (1975) Post-mortem changes in the chemistry and histology of normal and edematous brains. Amer J Path 79, 555–564

Hyperosmolar Solutions and Diuretics in the Treatment of Brain Edema

H. J. Klein and K. Schmidt

Introduction

Brain edema is the most common cause of increased intracranial pressure, whether restricted to a local area or occurring more diffusely. It is the uniform pathological reaction of brain tissue to disturbances of differing type and intensity. According to Klatzo [19] one must distinguish between a cytotoxic and a vasogenic edema. The questions regarding treatment of both types of edema are, therefore, naturally different. Cytotoxic edema results from a swelling of brain cells caused by a disturbance in energy supply, electrolyte regulation and inadequacy of the osmo-regulating processes. Vasogenic brain edema is characterized by an increased vascular permeability and disturbances of the blood brain barrier (BBB) which lead to permeation of proteins and other serum contents into the extracellular space.

Depending on the complexity of the pathophysiological consequences of brain edema there is a wide range of medical treatment with different mechanisms of action. When the brain edema causes an ICP exceeding 25–30 Hg, hyperosmolar solutions are used to lower this increased ICP.

This means that the optimal treatment of increased ICP has to be combined with the continuous recording of ICP. Therefore, in all those cases where we expect a markedly increased ICP we usually implant epidural ICP electrodes which makes continuous monitoring possible. Our experiences documented in this paper are based on a large series of continuous monitoring with the Gaeltec and the Ladd system, as well as discontinuous monitoring with intraventricular drainages [21].

Mechanism of Hyperosmolar Solutions in Brain Edema

The most important effect of this treatment is the reduction of intracranial pressure (ICP) by reduction of intracranial volume, not the reduction of brain edema itself (Fig. 1). The rapid intravenous infusion of hyperosmotic solutions leads to a hyperosmolarity of the serum, so that an osmotic gradient is built up to the extravascular space [1, 12]. This is dependent on the presence of a semipermeable membrane which restricts diffusion of hyperosmolar solution into the hypo-osmotic compartment. The lower the molecular weight of a substance the stronger is its effect as an osmotherapeutic agent, resulting in the absorption of increasing amounts of water. Furthermore, the slower the osmotherapeutic agent leaves the intravascular space, for instance, by renal excretion and the shorter the infusion time is the more effective is the osmotic gradient.

Treatment of Cerebral Edema
Edited by A. Hartmann and M. Brock

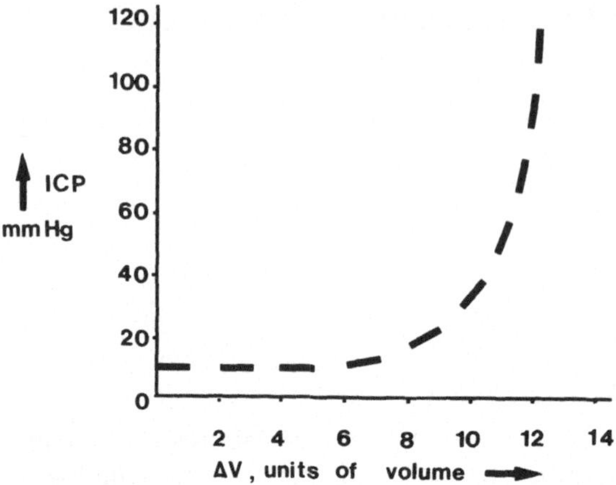

Fig. 1. Exponential volume/pressure relationship of intracranial pressure. Small amounts of additional volumes are compensated by reduction of cerebral blood flow and decreased production of cerebrospinal fluid. After the exhaustion of these mechanisms each additional unit of volume leads to a marked increase of intracranial pressure

The osmotic withdrawal of water depends on the intact BBB and does not function when disturbances of the barrier are present in cases of vasogenic edema, in contrast, there is a permeation of hypertonic solutions through the damaged barrier into the brain tissue, causing a rapid decline of the osmotic acting gradients. Such gradients will not be constituted in the first place by osmotherapy.

The decrease in ICP depends mainly on the reduction of normal brain tissue volume, which means that there is an osmotic withdrawal of water from the extravascular space into the vascular compartment. Since cytotoxic brain edema is mostly an intracellular damage which is not linked with severe blood brain barrier alterations, we expect a certain effectiveness in the case of cytotoxic brain edema [32]. An example for the successful reduction of ICP by osmotherapy is the volume reduction of healthy brain areas, which are clearly larger than the edematous compartment with its BBB disturbance. We expect this treatment to fail in general edema, especially in vasogenic edema with its particularly pronounced BBB disturbance [21].

What Causes the Increase of Pressure Above the Initial Level After Osmotherapy (the so Called Rebound Effect)?

The permeation of hyperosmotic solutions through the altered BBB can lead to an increased effusion into the edematous compartment, resulting in an increased volume. This leads to corresponding ICP increase (rebound effect), if the volume increase of the edema exceeds the volume reduction of the healthy brain compartment (Fig. 2). An increased water congestion in the edematous compartment is not only favoured by the permeation of the hyperosmotic solution, but also by the fact, that there is mainly water – but no significant sodium excretion. Thus, this sodium retention will cause a renewed hydration [27]. This phenomenon is also the reason for a partial rehydration after osmotherapy in cases of cytotoxic edema.

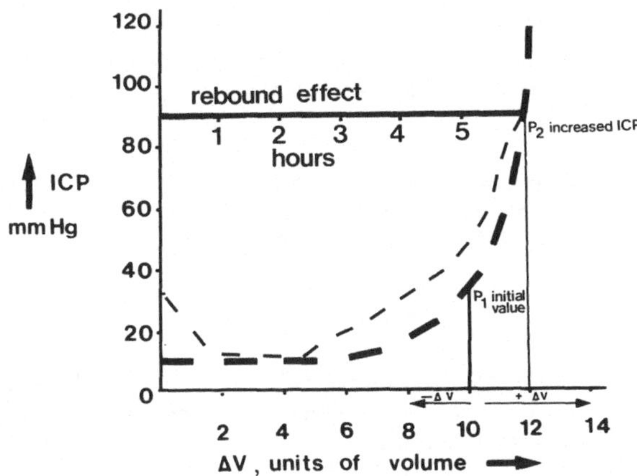

Fig. 2. The rebound effect in terms of the exponential volume/pressure relationship. If the volume increase of the edema caused by permeation of hypertonic solutions exceeds the volume reduction of the healthy brain compartment (+delta V larger than − delta V) a pressure increase following osmotherapy can be observed

The reduction in brain pressure declines when there is an elimination or reversal of osmotic gradient by rapid metabolism or excretion and fluid expansion in the vascular compartment. In spite of the increase in ICP which may near the initial level, but not exceed it, as the pressure inducing edema still exists, one should not speak of the rebound effect before the initial value is exceeded. The literature concerning the frequency of the rebound effect differs considerably, reaching from some few percent up to 31.8% [3]. Reulen [27] expects the rebound effect in all cases of osmotherapy for post-traumatic brain edema. According to Hase and Reulen [14] no rebound effect will occur when the pressure-inducing edema can be permanently lowered to a lower level by hyperosmotic-induced pressure reduction. The causes can be found especially in the increase of CBF and the reduction of lactacidosis. This means that osmotherapy does not primarily reduce the edema, but influences the edema-propagating factors in decreasing the ICP.

Additional Mechanisms Caused by Hypertonic Solutions

Besides the desirable effect of reducing the volume of the intracranial contents and the corresponding ICP, an osmotic induced increase of plasma volume leads to a reduction of blood viscosity (Fig. 3) and peripheral arterial resistance, resulting in an increase of the mean arterial blood pressure, stroke volume and the oxygen transport capacity [33, 35, 36, 38]. A longer lasting decrease of ICP caused by dehydration of brain tissue raises the intracranial perfusion pressure and the CBF. Occasionally there is an initial increase of ICP. This paradoxical reaction is caused by an increase in stroke volume and consecutive CBF elevation before the dehydration lowers the ICP. As the result of reduced ICP, there will also be improved circulation in areas with insufficient perfusion which so far have no vasogenic edema (border line). The favorable rheological attributes of osmotherapy persists only during the

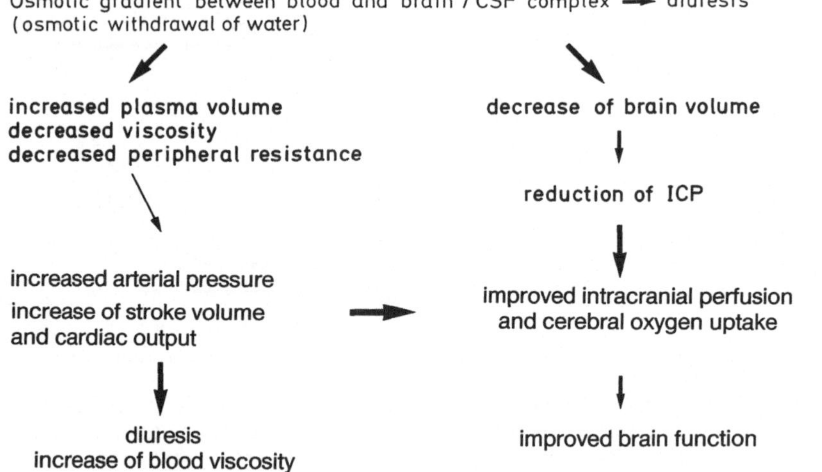

Fig. 3. Mechanism of action of hypertonic solutions on increased ICP

phase of osmotic induced withdrawal of water from the extravascular space. After this, there will be a phase of augmented diuresis and metabolism, so that these favorable hemodynamic factors once again become worse [38]. For this reason it is necessary to maintain these favorable rheological and hemodynamic factors by further infusions of albumin or other osmotic agents (Fig. 3).

Side-Effects of Osmotherapy

Osmotherapy leads to a more or less pronounced dehydration. The danger of over-dehydration becomes greater when the mobilized water having been drawn from the extracellular space is eliminated by an induced increase in diuresis. In this way a significant loss of water would result. By repeated osmotherapy the osmolarity of tissue increases by dehydration and partial diffusion of the agent itself, resulting in the decrease of the osmotic gradient, of the effectivity and of the duration. Theoretically, this gradient could be maintained by a continued hyperosmosis with solutions at an increased absolute level. Osmolarity values above 320 mosmol/kg induce an osmotic opening of the BBB (tight junctions), thus increasing a tendency towards edema. At the same time the dangers of osmotically induced brain edema and of osmotic nephrosis by increased sodium concentrations will grow [5, 7, 42].

Clinical Experiences with Hypertonic Solutions

There are sufficient clinical and experimental results during the last two decades to demonstrate the usefulness of hyperosmotic sorbitol and mannitol infusions [9, 33, 34, 41, 45].

Table 1. Pharmacological effects of hyperosmolar solutions

%	Substance	Molecular weight	Usual dosage (g/kg/body weight)	Duration of ICP reduction (hours)	Duration of stroke volume increase (hours)	Increased diuresis	Metabolic utilisation	Renal excretion	Rebound phenomenon	Side effects
30	Urea	62	1.0	6	3/4	+ + +	–	–	+ +	Disorders of haemostasis
15	Glycerine	90	0.5	2	1	+	+	+	+	Haemolysis tubulusnecrosis
50	Glucose	180	0.5	3/4	3/4	–	+	+	+	Insulin-dependent utilisation
40	Laevulose	180	1.5	2	1	+	+	+	+	–
40	Sorbitol	182	1.5	2.5	1	+	+	+	+	Contraindicated in fructose intolerance
15	Mannitol	182	1.5	+6	1.5	+ +	–	+	+	Dehydration

Table 2. Comparison of various factors after infusions of hyperosmolar solutions and after ventricular drainage

CBF Measurement (Kety-Schmidt method)	40 min after infusion of 250 cm³ sorbitol –40% – in 20 min. iv. $n=6$ (K. Schmidt)			30 min after infusion of 150 cm³ glucose –50% – Rapid dosage iv. $n=6$ (Shenkin et al.)			30 min after CSF withdrawal –Ventricular drainage – $n=6$ (Shenkin et al.)		
	$\bar{X}$%		$P<$	$\bar{X}$%		$P<$	$\bar{X}$%		$P<$
1. Cerebral blood flow	+44.34	±189.0	0.001	+24.7	±27.2	0.1	+ 6.2	±6.6	0.1
2. Oxygen uptake	+24.58	± 24.8	0.05	+12.1	±17.5	0.2	+ 3.3	±4.9	0.05
3. Cerebral vascular resistance	–23.25	± 16.2	0.02	–20.8	±17.3	0.05	– 7.3	±6.9	0.05
4. CSF pressure	–82.0			–47.0			–72.0		

Sorbitol 40% has an osmolality of 3,219 mosmol/kg body weight and, therefore, a strong effect on reducing ICP. It is not only excreted by the kidneys, but rapidly metabolized to a great extent over the fructose utilization pathway. After rapid injection its presence can no longer be detected after an hour [13]. The intracranial pressure reduction lasts between one and three hours (Table 2). Mannitol 15% or 20% has a somewhat less marked effect which takes longer to become active, but lasts. Even after six hours it can still be detected in the serum, as mannitol is only excreted by the kidneys (Table 1).
Some characteristics of osmotherapy can be deduced from the above mentioned results which have been elaborated on and proved by numerous authors [4, 8, 9, 14, 15, 27, 33, 35, 41],

1. the *rate* of infusion of osmotherapeutic agents determines the *degree* of ICP reduction,
2. the *amount* of the infusion determines the *duration* of ICP reduction,
3. sorbitol has a stronger but shorter lasting effect than mannitol (at the same rate of infusion),
4. small quantities of these solutions rapidly injected (e.g. 50–80 cc sorbitol or 100–150 cc mannitol in 5 to 10 minutes) are also sufficient in cases of acute ICP increases, without problems of increased osmolality and electrolyte disturbances; for,
5. at a high initial ICP only small doses of hypertonic solutions are needed, as small changes in volume cause great changes in pressure according to the exponential volume pressure relationship (Fig. 1),
6. accordingly a large quantity of hyperosmotic solutions is necessary at gradually increased pressure in order to reach additional ICP reduction (Fig. 1).

Certain Indications for Osmotherapy

Osmotherapy is absolutely necessary in cases of acute herniation [31] and marked increase of ICP. A potent osmotherapeutic agent (40% sorbitol) should be quickly injected in less than five minutes at a dose of 0.5–0.7 g/kg body weight, after which a mannitol infusion should be given. The favorable influence on critical ICP increase by means of osmotherapy should be used taking all operative measures to prevent an additional increase in CSF pressure, if an operative procedure can eliminate the cause of brain edema and ICP (removal of space occupying hematoma or tumor, ventricular drainage or shunt operation) [18, 20, 35]. For further procedures the following facts must be considered:

1. ICP reduction is of limited duration,
2. there may be a rebound effect with renewed increase of ICP, even above the initial level,
3. in acute and chronic intracranial hematoma renewed bleeding occupying additional space, can be provoked which may lead to increased ICP when the osmotherapeutical effect has ended,
4. the ICP decrease can be smaller in cases of pronounced atrophy (e.g. hydrocephalus) due to the limited possibilities of withdrawing water when compared to the

amount of tissue in a normal sized brain. In addition all compensating mechanisms in chronic ICP are frequently used up, so that small increases in volume critically reduce the intracranial perfusion pressure.

Mannitol (15%) 0.7–1.5 g/kg bodyweight is the average dose for marked increases of ICP. Also, there are results confirmed by ICP monitoring which show the effectiveness of small repeated doses in reducing ICP values exceeding 250–300 mm H_2O in order to bridge the gap of the critical phase of threatened herniation [14].
As Table 1 shows, mannitol has the longest lasting ICP reducing effect of all used osmotherapeutic agents in comparatively long plasma expansion and stroke volume increase. Mannitol is especially appropriate for the preparation of neurosurgical operations [27, 39, 40]. Mannitol infusions *before* narcosis ensure a long-lasting reduction of ICP during the operation and improved hemodynamic conditions even with the introduction of narcosis and its possible effect on the stability of circulation. After craniotomy and opening of the dura mater, the hemodynamic effect has already stopped while ICP lowering still continues, so that increased bleeding and brain congestion caused by an possible initial paradoxical reaction by plasma expansion and increased CBF need no longer be feared.

What Can Osmotherapy Not Achieve?

As earlier mentioned, osmotherapy will cause no reduction of ICP when the volume increase due to permeation of osmotic acting agents into the damaged brain area is larger than the volume reduction of the remaining healthy brain tissue (Fig. 2). In the presence of space occupying lesions such as tumors or hematomas ICP lowering infusions of hypertonic solutions can only have the gap-bridging effect until the necessary operative treatment starts [20].
Long lasting treatment with sorbitol as the hypertonic solution does not exist, as the rapid metabolism of sorbitol only brings about a nutritional effect, without constituting an effective osmotic gradient [13]. A possible indication for long lasting therapy with mannitol should be discussed.

New Indications for Osmotherapy

Miller and Leech [23] came to the conclusion that mannitol reduces the pressure volume index earlier and more markedly than the ICP itself. This means that ICP reacts less to additional volume rates, making it appear that mannitol fulfils a double function as regards the reduction of ICP. Because of the additional favorable characteristics of mannitol, independent of its hyperosmotic action to influence positively the volume pressure quotient, also called "compliance", we now understand the efficacy of forms of treatment practiced by James [2, 17] and Brown et al.
The continuous infusion of mannitol contradicts the principle of quickly establishing the hyperosmolarity of the blood. However, James [17] showed in a series of continuous mannitol infusions, which were given to 18 patients, that in 16 cases the ICP could be significantly reduced. In the course of 24 hours 4–5 g/kg body weight

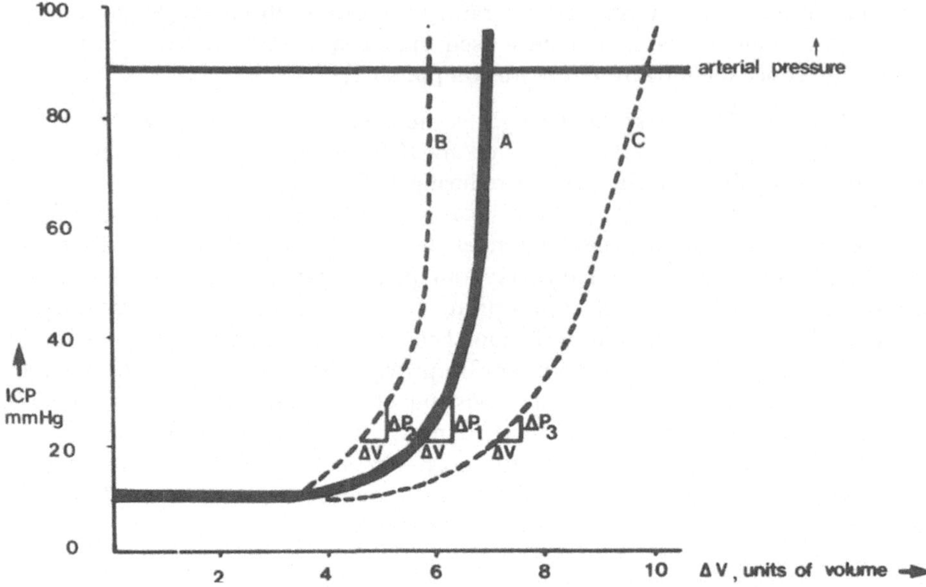

Fig. 4. Relation between intracranial volume and intracranial pressure under various conditions [23]. *A* normal relation; *B* curve in patients with arterial hypertension may shift to the left; *C* mannitol renders the intracranial contents more tolerant to a volume addition

was continuously injected. The osmolarity of the serum had values between 276 and 301 mosmol/l, more favourable than in bolus injections with values between 276 and 354 mosmol/l. When mannitol is injected quickly it effects the volume pressure quotient and has the well-known hyperosmotic effects; whereas the continuous infusion of mannitol only appears to reduce the ICP by improvement of "compliance" (Fig. 4).

The resulting consequences for treatment are as follows: a continuous mannitol infusion can be given when the ICP does not exceed a pressure of 250–300 mm H_2O. In acute pressure increases, that is in cases with a pressure of more than 400 mm H_2O, a bolus injection should be given by eventual continuous infusions.

Optimal Osmotherapy by ICP Monitoring

In this context we should collect clinical experiences supported by ICP monitoring with bolus injections of small amounts of sorbitol and continuous injections of mannitol at the same time. The strongest increases in ICP with critical phases of herniation syndromes occur primarily in severe head injuries with extensive brain contusions. Here it is definitely advantageous, almost necessary in some complicated cases, to make osmotherapy dependent on continuous ICP monitoring because there can be an enormous dissociation between the clinical picture and associated ICP. Furthermore small amounts of sorbitol can be given at shorter intervals than six hours which had been recommended previously. ICP monitoring can exactly determine the necessary frequency of osmotherapeutical administrations and it has been suggested that ICP control during repeated mannitol administrations can only be achieved at osmolarity levels which are tolerated on a long-term basis (310 mosm or less) because each manitol administration raises the serum osmolarity.

Prophylaxis for Brain Edema. Does it Exist?

Concerning this question we have to distinguish exactly between the different etiology and types of edema. It must be stressed that it is preferable to maintain the colloid osmotic pressure at the optimal level (approximately 30 mosmol/kg H_2O) because this figure is responsible for resorption of interstitial fluid at the venous end of the capillaries. This can be obtained by the above mentioned infusions of albumin solutions. The colloid osmotic pressure drops as a result of diluting albumin in those cases which have not received infusions of osmotic agents (Figs. 5, 6) (Tullis [44], Klein [21]).

Edema prophylaxis seems to be reasonable when a decrease in CBF caused by vascular lesions is feared. There are clinical and experimental results which show that mannitol infusions can prevent ICP increases caused by edema especially in the case of vasogenic edema [2, 24]. In addition we have had the clinical experience that external ventricular drainage can be removed without additional lumbar punctures, by giving continuous infusions of mannitol.

In conclusion we want to mention the prophylaxis of edema with mannitol in the treatment of cerebral ischemia. In cases of strokes of varying intensity without hemorrhagic infarctions the infusion of mannitol has proved to be effective. This treatment is combined with the infusion of oncotic agents like rheomacrodex or albumin solutions [10, 11, 16].

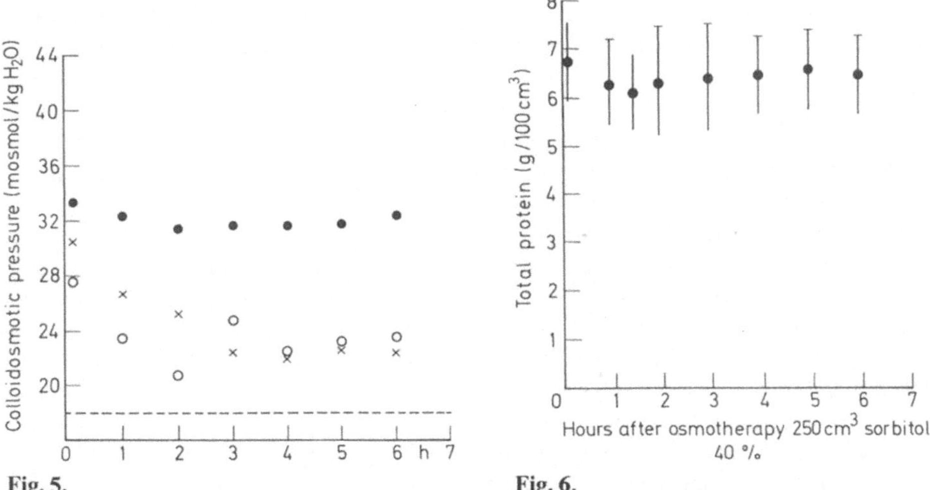

Fig. 5.

Fig. 6.

Fig. 5. Colloidal osmotic pressure after infusion of 750 ccm 15% mannitol over min

Fig. 6. Decrease of total protein serum after osmotherapy with 250 ccm 40% sorbitol. N = 10 patients. Maximum decrease after 90 min of osmotherapy

Furthermore we used to give continuous infusions of mannitol to all those patients suffering from arterial spasm due to subarachnoid hemorrhage who receive treatment by induced hypertension with dopamine infusions. In these cases the continuous infusion of mannitol renders the intracranial contents more tolerant to a volume addition caused by intracranial blood volume and counteracts directly the negative influence of arterial hypertension ([2, 23], Van der Werf, personal communication 1981) (Fig. 4).

Experiences with Computer Tomographic Control of Patients After Therapy with Hypertonic Solutions

Although the cranial computer tomography is an excellent method [22] to demonstrate the cerebral edema in man we failed to show any change in densities in computer tomography of patients which had been treated with hypertonic solutions even during the time when a maximal decrease of ICP was noted.

There was only a distinct difference in the densities after treatment with hypertonic solution when this agent was administered to a healthy person who had a normal cranial computer tomogram (Fig. 7).

Experiences with Diuretics in Treatment of Brain Edema

Investigations made in animals, which prove the efficacy of frusemide, acetazolamide, have shown some conflicting and divergent results. Principally there is no added effect when these substances are combined with mannitol, nor has the combination of two diuretics shown an increased effect [18].

The treatment of brain edema with diuretics is based on the fact that a dehydration with a negative waterbalance leads to a general dehydration of body tissue fluid, and on the fact that the developing brain edema is characterized by increased sodium and water retention [28].

Nevertheless, there is no general agreement concerning the efficacy of diuretics in reducing brain edema. Meinig [25, 26] found a reduction of edema, especially of the perifocal type, when he treated brain tumor patients with a combination therapy of dexamethasone and frusemide. Also treatment with etacrynacid, extending over several days, was capable of causing a distinct reduction of brain edema in brain tumor patients [30]. Recently reports have been written about the pharmacological action of diuretics, postulating a brain pressure reducing effect by lowering the CSF secretion rate [29]. There are also results which have proved the theory, that the active transport of sodium to brain tissue and the CSF spaces is blocked, a theory which is also supported by Sklar [43]. Richard [32] found a reduction rate of ICP of 20–40% of the initial level in 40–50% of his patients, treated with frusemide. In this study a very delayed maximum reduction of ICP (after six hours) was recorded.

Diuretics induce a negative water balance and an increased hemoconcentration thus rendering decreased cerebral microcirculation. Furthermore we have to reflect that brain edema is caused by a local BBB disturbance and not by general overhydration. The favorable rheological and hemodynamic effects which we can expect after

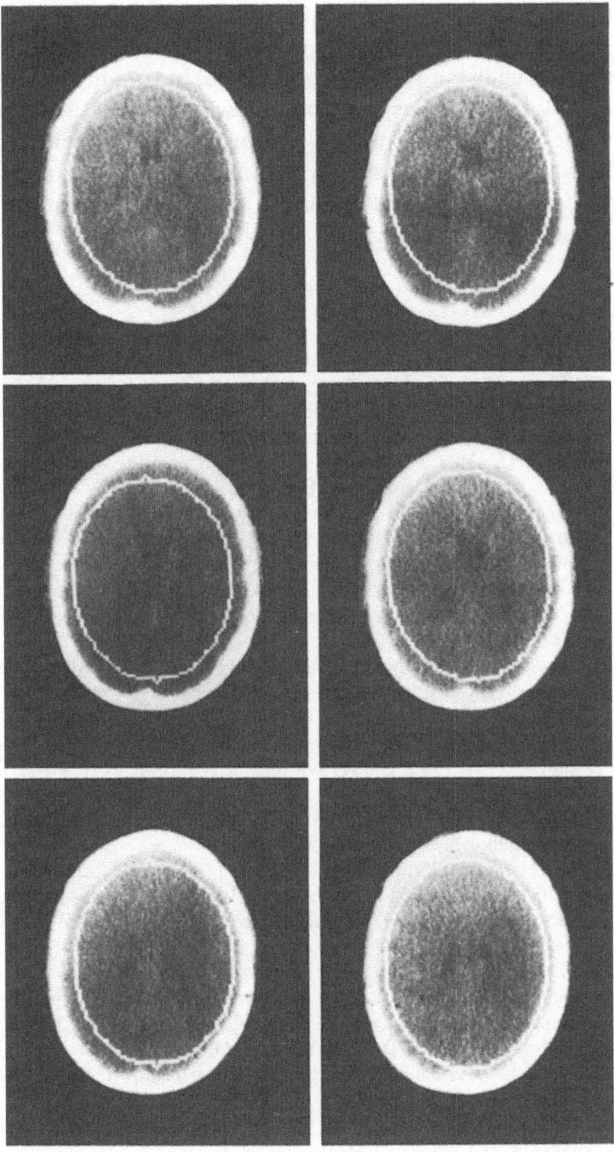

Fig. 7. Computer tomography before (*left*) and after (*right*) mannitol infusion (750 ml, 15%) in a volunteer doctor. The increase in density from 34–35, respectively from 33–35 and from 34–36 would result from the withdrawal of interstitial fluid

treatment with osmotic and oncotic acting agents cannot be seen after treatment with diuretics [37].

Various studies concerning patients with head injuries, and experimental work based on induced cold lesions proved that the rate of reduction of ICP by diuretics is smaller than the rate reached with hyperosmolar solutions. In many cases there was no diuretic induced reduction of pressure at all [6, 8]. These authors concluded that the only rational use is in the combination therapy with dexamethasone which reduces the peritumoral edema. Eventually, a low dosage following hypertonic solutions extends the ICP reducing phase, but we must stress that each single infusion of hypertonic solutions must be followed by oncotic acting volumes to prevent a general exsiccosis, for merely the infusion of therapeutical dosages of hypertonic solutions will cause a considerable reduction in the content of water in the extravascular space (depending on the dosage of sorbitol or mannitol exceeding 1000 ccm) which is not linked with diuresis.

References

1. Bürger M (1925) Über Osmotherapie. Ther Gegenw 27:27–30, 72–75
2. Brown FD, Hanlon K, Mullan SM (1978) Treatment of aneurysmal hemiplegia with dopamine and mannitol. J Neurosurg 49:525–529
3. Ferrer E, Vila F, Isamaat F (1980) Mannitol response and histogram analysis in raised ICP. In: ICP IV, Springer, Berlin Heidelberg New York, pp 647–652
4. Gaab M, Knoblich OE, Schupp J, Dietrich K, Fuhrmeister U, Gruss P (1978) Wirkung unterschiedlicher Osmo- und Onkotherapie auf Hirndruck und elektrische Hirnaktivität beim experimentellen Hirnödem. Acta Neurochir 40, 203–221
5. Gaab M, Pflughaupt KW, Ratzka M, Wodarz R, Gruss P (1978) Critical intracranial effects of osmotherapy. Advances in Neurosurgery, vol 6. Springer, Berlin Heidelberg New York, pp 193–205
6. Gaab M, Knoblich OE, Schupp J, Hermann F, Fuhrmeister U, Pflughaupt KW (1979) Effects of frusemide (Lasix) on acute severe experimental cerebral edema. J Neurol 220, 185–192
7. Gaab M, Trost HA, Haubitz I, Pflughaupt KW, Halves E (1980) Osmoregulation, Brain damage and Prognosis. Advances in Neurosurgery, vol 8. Springer, Berlin Heidelberg New York
8. Gaab M, Bushe KA (1981) Die Behandlung der intrakraniellen Drucksteigerung. Intensivbehandlung 6:1, 34–52
9. Goluboff B, Shenkin HA, Haft H (1964) The effects of mannitol and urea on cerebral hemodynamics and cerebrospinal fluid pressure. Neurology (Minneap) 14, 891–898
10. Gottstein U (1974) Behandlung der cerebralen Mangeldurchblutung. Internist 15, 575–587
11. Gottstein U (1977) personal communication
12. Hagemann E (1920) Über osmotische Wirkungen intravenöser Zuckerinjektionen unter wechselnden Bedingungen. Zschr Ges Exp Med 11, 239–256
13. Halmágyi M (1970) Veränderungen des Wasser- und Elektrolythaushaltes durch Osmotherapie. Anaesthesiology and Resuscitation, vol 46, Springer, Berlin Heidelberg New York
14. Hase U, Reulen HJ (1980) Wirkung von Sorbit und Mannit auf den intrakraniellen Druck. Neurochirurgia 23, 205–211
15. Hermann F, Gaab M, Pflughaupt KW, Gruss P (1981) Medikamentöse Therapie beim experimentellen Hirnödem. Neurochirurgica 24, 39–46
16. Herrschaft H (1976) Die Therapie der cerebralen Mangeldurchblutung. Der Nervenarzt 47, 639–650
17. James HE (1980) Methodology for the control of intracranial pressure with hypertonic mannitol. In: ICP IV, Springer, Berlin Heidelberg New York, pp 653–655
18. James HE, Harbaugh RD, Marshall LF, Shapiro HM, Laurin R (1980) The response to multiple therapeutic modalities in experimental vasogenic edema. In: ICP IV, Springer, Berlin Heidelberg New York, pp 272–276
18. Isfort A (1966) Indikationen der Osmotherapie in der Neurochirurgie. In: Anaesthesiologie und Wiederbelebung. Bd. 13: Infusionstherapie. Springer, Berlin Heidelberg New York

19. Klatzo I, Wisniewski H, Steinwall O, Steicher E (1967) Dynamics of cold injury edema. In: Brain edema. Klatzo, Seitelberger (eds). Springer, Berlin Heidelberg New York, pp 554–563
20. Klein HJ (1980) Gedeckte Schädel-Hirn-Traumen. Notfallmedizin 6, 860–872
21. Klein HJ (1982) Kontinuierliche Hirndruckregistrierung – Teil jeder Hirndrucktherapie? Klinikarzt 5, 520–527
22. Lanksch W, Grumme Th, Kazner E (1978) Schädelhirnverletzungen im Computertomogramm. Springer, Berlin Heidelberg New York
23. Leech P, Miller JD (1975) The effect of mannitol, steroids and hypocapnia on the intracranial volume/pressure response. In: ICP II. Springer, Berlin Heidelberg New York, pp 301–364
24. Little J (1978) Modification of acute focal ischemia by treatment with mannitol and high-dose dexamethasone. J Neurosurg 49, 517–524
25. Meinig G, Aulich A, Wende S, Reulen HJ (1976) The effects of dexamethasone and diuretics on peritumor brain edema: Comparative study of tissue water content and CT. In: Dynamics of brain edema. Pappius HM, Feindl W (eds). Springer, Berlin Heidelberg New York, pp 301–305
26. Meinig G (1980) Beurteilung der antiödematösen Therapie bei Hirntumorpatienten. Neurochirurgia 23, 212–218
27. Reulen HJ (1965) Vor- und Nachteile der osmotischen Behandlung des Hirnödems. Zbl Neurochir 26:4/5, 232–249
28. Reulen HJ, Medzihradsky F, Enzenbach R, Marguth F, Brendel W (1969) Electrolytes, fluids, and energy metabolism in human cerebral edema. Arch Neurol 21, 517–525
29. Reulen HJ (1976) Vasogenic brain oedema. New aspects in its formation, resolution and therapy. Br J Anaesth 48:741–752
30. Reulen HJ, Steude U, Brendel W, Hilber C, Prusiner S (1970) Energetische Störungen des Kationentransports als Ursache des intrazellulären Hirnödems. Acta Neurochir 22, 129–166
31. Reulen HJ, Schürmann K (1981) Nonsurgical management of severe head injuries. Prog neurol Surg, vol 10, 291–322, Karger, Basel
32. Richard KE (1980) Intrakranielle Drucksteigerung, ihre Pathogenese, Klinik und Behandlung. Nervenarzt 51, 392–405
33. Schmidt K (1963) Zur Wirkung einiger Osmotherapeutika. Anaesthesist 12, 216–222
34. Schmidt K (1966) Zur Behandlung von Hirndruck und Hirnödem in der Neurochirurgie und in der Unfallchirurgie durch Osmo- und Onkotherapie. Schlesw-Holst Ärztebl 18:7
35. Schmidt K (1966) Klinisch-experimentelle Grundlagen der Osmotherapie. In: Anaesthesiologie und Wiederbelebung, Bd. 13: Infusionstherapie. Springer, Berlin Göttingen
36. Schmidt K, Schmalz H (1967) Zur Blutvolumenänderung nach Osmo-Onko-Therapie. Anaesthesist 16:201–204
37. Schmidt K (1967) Zur Onkotherapie des Hirnödems mit Furosemid. Acta Neurochirurgica 17, 32
38. Schmidt K (1970) Einfluß der Plasmaviskositätsänderungen nach Osmo- und Onkotherapie auf die Hämodynamik. Anaesthesist 19, 146–152
39. Schmidt K (1972) Hirndurchblutung bei intrakranieller Drucksteigerung und beim Hirnödem. In: Der Hirnkreislauf. Physiologie–Pathologie–Klinik. Gänshirt H (ed). Thieme, Stuttgart
40. Schultis K, Gofferje H, Brand O (1976) Zur Osmotherapie im zentrogenen Schock. In Neurogener Schock. Schattauer, Stuttgart, pp 83–89
41. Shenkin HA, Goluboff B, Haft H (1962) The use of mannitol for the reduction of ICP in intracranial surgery. J Neurosurg 19, 897–901
42. Silber SJ, Thompson N (1972) Mannitol induced central nervous system toxicity in renal failure. Invest Urol 9, 310–312
43. Sklar FH, Beyer CW Jr, Ramanathan M, Clark WK (1980) The effects of frusemide on CSF dynamics in patients with pseudotumor cerebri. In: ICP IV. Springer, Berlin Heidelberg New York, pp 660–663
44. Tullis JL (1977) Albumin 1. Background and Use. JAMA Vol 237:4:355–360
45. Wise BL, Chater N (1962) The value of hypertonic mannitol solutions in decreasing brain mass and lowering cerebrospinal fluid pressure. J Neurosurg 19, 1038–1043

The Effect of High Doses of Steroids on Traumatic Brain Edema

W. Gobiet

Introduction

The aim of our study was to evaluate the effect of high doses of dexamethasone on acute cerebral edema. The work was performed in two parts. A pilot study on 93 patients with head injuries was followed by an open study, which included 672 patients. The latter lasted over four years.

1. Pilot Study

The patients were divided in three groups: Group I did not receive any dexamethasone, group II received a dose of 16 mg initially, followed by 4 mg every 6 hours, group III received high doses of dexamethasone (48 mg initially, 8 mg every two hours).
All patients had suffered from a closed head injury. They were comatose at time of admittance with aimless reaction to painful stimuli. At least one pupil reacted to light.
Intracranial pressure (ICP) was measured by an epidural device.
Treatment was standardized: it consisted of mild hyperventilation, high calorie nutrition and maintenance of blood homeostasis. All patients received hypertonic solutions (1 g/kg body wt) when ICP exceeded 50 mm Hg.

Results

Table 1 summarizes the incidence of pressure rises within the groups. It became obvious that in group III (high dose) increases of ICP beyond 25 mm Hg were sig-

Table 1. Incidence of highest intracranial pressure levels in all groups

ICP (mm Hg)	Group		
	I	II	III
0 – 25	6	3	22
25 – 50	3	4	2
> 50	26	16	10

Treatment of Cerebral Edema
Edited by A. Hartmann and M. Brock

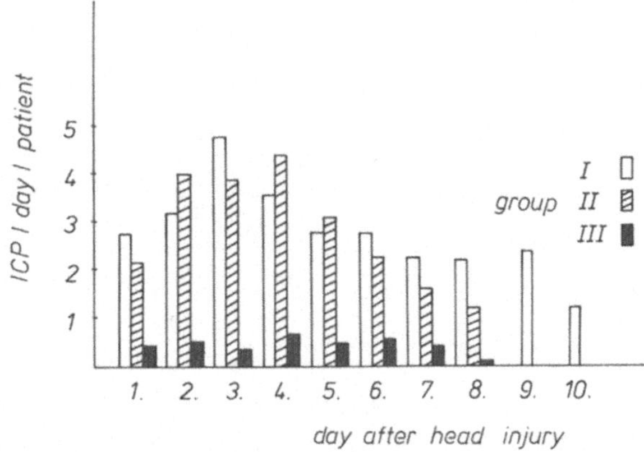

Fig. 1. Frequency of pathological increases in pressure within all groups. I: control group. II: low dose dexamethasone. III: high dose dexamethasone

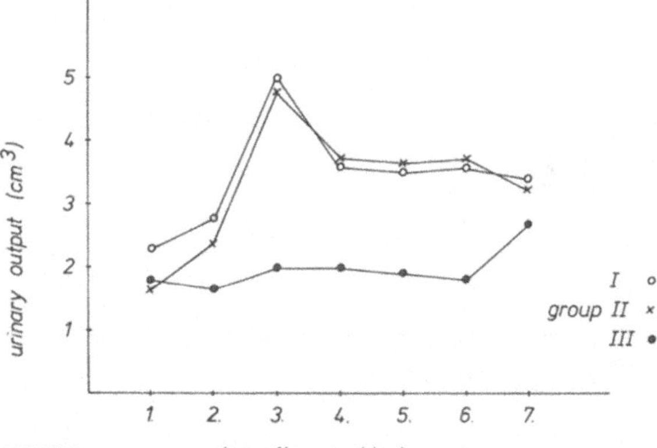

Fig. 2. Average urinary output in all groups

nificantly less frequent than in the other two groups. To compare the effect of dexamethasone directly among the three groups the total number of ICP increases over 50 mm Hg for each post-traumatic day were added within the group and then divided by the number of patients. Figure 1 shows the result of this analysis.

In groups I and II the numbers of pathological increases of ICP over 50 mm Hg were almost equal. In the group with a high dose of dexamethasone (III) they were significantly lower. As a result patients in group I and II needed more hypertonic solutions than those in group III to lower the ICP below the critical level of 50 mm Hg.

In groups I and II urinary output was markedly greater than in those patients who received high doses of steroids (Fig. 2).

Average serum osmolarity increased to the critical level of 340 mosm/l on the first to third post-traumatic days in groups I and II whereas in group III it remained in a normal range over the whole period of observation (Fig. 3). Electrolytes and blood sugar levels were almost the same in all groups.

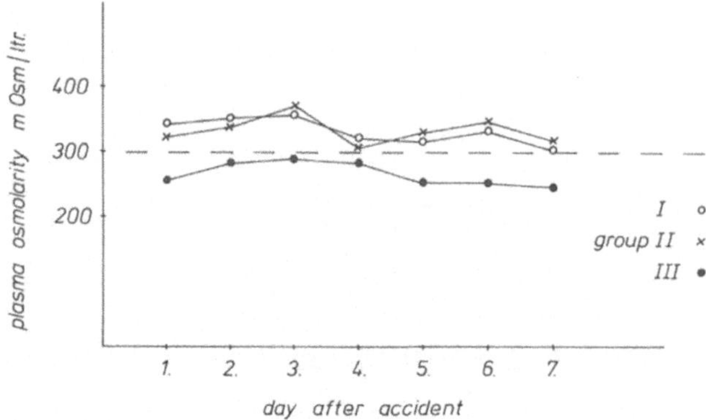

Fig. 3. Serum osmolarity in all groups

Table 2. Rate of mortality and of complications in all groups

No. of patients	Group I	Group II	Group III
	35	24	34
Died	45.5%	41.5%	23%
Pulmonary edema	7	4	0
Gastric hemorrhage	5	3	0

The mortality rate decreased significantly from 45% and 47% in groups I and II to 23% in group III (Table 2).

2. Open Study

Encouraged by these results a second study was performed, which lasted from 1972–1976.

From 1972–1974 none of the patients with head injuries who were admitted to the intensive careunit unit of the neurosurgical department of the University of Essen (Dir.: Prof. Dr. Grote) received any steroids.

In 1975 and 1976 all patients received high doses of dexamethasone (100 mg initially, 8 mg every 3 hours). The average age ranged about 28 years in adults and nine years in children. Duration of unconsciousness (Fig. 4) and type of injury was about equal in the two groups (Fig. 5). Prophylaxis and therapy of brain edema was as nearly similar as possible (Table 3).

The results showed a significantly lower mortality in the high dose group (Table 4). It decreased in adults from 55% to 38% and in children from 42–15.6%.

The quality of the outcome was significantly better for patients in the group with the high doses. In the children 62% (90%) were full work or school against 40% (75%) in the first group.

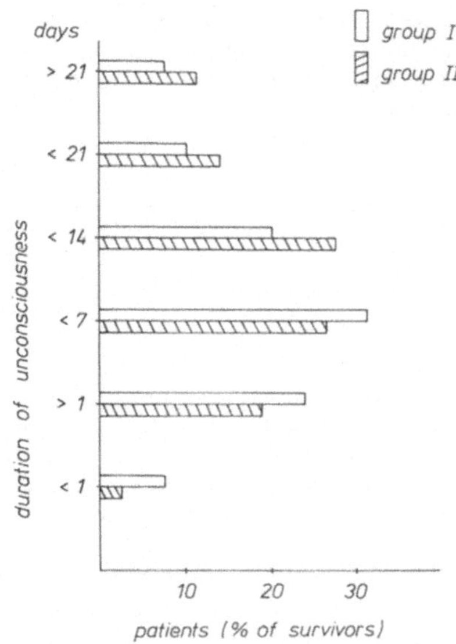

Fig. 4. Duration of unconsciousness in relationship to percentage of surviving patients

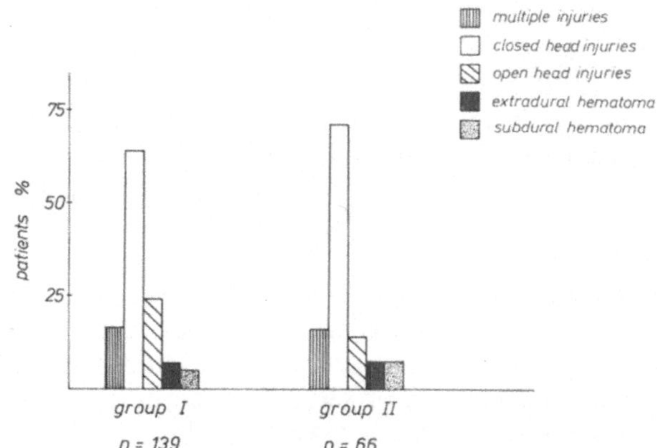

Fig. 5. Type of injury in both groups of the open study

Table 3. Basic therapy in both groups (brain edema)

Prophylaxis	Treatment
Clear the airway	
Hyperventilation	Hypertonic solution (1 g/kg/bw) if:
Balanced infusion therapy	ICP above 50 mm Hg
High Calorie nutrition	CPP below 50 mm Hg
High doses of dexamethasone	

Table 4. Mortality and clinical outcome in the open study. From 1972 till 1974 none of the patients admitted received any steroids. From 1975 – 1976 all patients with closed head injury received dexamethasone 100 mg initally and thereafter 8 mg every 3 hours. In this group mortality was lower

	Adults > 14 years	Children < 14 years
1972 – 1974		
Mortality	285 (55%)	114 (42%)
Unconscious stabilized	6 patients	4 patients
At work or school	40%	75%
1975 – 1976		
Mortality	177 (38%)	96 (15.6%)
Unconscious stabilized	4 patients	2 patients
At work or school	62%	90%

Only 4 (2) patients remained unconscious three months after injury whereas 6 (4) patients developed an apallic syndrome in the "no steroid" group.

In spite of complications, electrolyte and blood sugar disturbances were equal. The rate of pulmonary infection was slightly higher in the high dose group. No patient developed signs of adrenal gland insufficiency.

Discussion

Many investigations report a positive effect of steroid in the treatment of perifocal edema in cases of brain tumors [1, 7, 8]. On the other hand any favorable effect [2] of dexamethasone in acute brain injury is denied by some authors. Thus the administration of osmo-diuretics remains the preferred treatment of post-traumatic cerebral edema [6].

According to our experience, osmotherapy has proved insufficient to prevent or successfully treat cerebral edema associated with severe head injury. Limitations for this therapy were urinary outputs over 5 litres/day with the risk of progressive dehydration, and increase of serum osmolarity over the critical level of 340 mosm/l. Thus we were not able to lower mortality significantly in the untreated group or in the group treated with normal doses of dexamethasone. Comparing the results of the different groups, dexamethasone showed a direct dose-dependent effect on ICP [4, 5]. Only very high doses were able to reduce significantly the number of pathologic increases in ICP, whereas the commonly recommended low doses of this drug showed no therapeutic effect on ICP as compared with the group not receiving dexamethasone.

Since the mortality rate also dropped significantly and the clinical outcome was better, high doses of dexamethasone must be recommended as basic treatment, especially in younger patients, to prevent traumatic brain edema [3, 5].

References

1. Brock M (1976) The effect of dexamethasone on intracranial pressure in patients with supratentorial tumors. Dynamics of brain edema. Springer, Berlin Heidelberg New York, pp 330–336
2. Faupel G, Reulen HJ, Müller D, Schürmann K (1976) Double-blind study on the effects of steroids on severe closed head injury. Dynamics of brain edema. Springer, Berlin Heidelberg New York, pp 337–343
3. Gobiet W (1976) The influence of various doses of dexamethasone on intracranial pressure in patients with severe head injury. Dynamics of brain edema. Springer, Berlin Heidelberg New York, pp 351–356
4. Gobiet W, Bock WJ, Liesegang J, Grote W (1974) Experience with an intracranial pressure transducer, readjustable in vivo. J Neurosurg 40, 272–276
5. Gobiet W, Grote W, Bock WJ (1975) The relation between intracranial pressure, mean arterial pressure and cerebral blood flow in patients with severe head injury. Acta Neurochir (Wien) 32, 13–24
6. Kühner A (1973) The influence of high and low dosages of mannitol 25% in the therapy of cerebral edema. In: Brain edema. Vol I, Springer, Berlin Heidelberg New York
7. Reulen HJ, Hadjidimos A (1973) Steroids in the treatment of brain edema. In: Brain edema. Vol I, Springer, Berlin Heidelberg New York
8. Reulen HJ, Schürmann K (1972) Steroids and brain edema. Springer, Berlin Heidelberg New York

The Effect of Dexamethasone on the Level of Adrenaline and Noradrenaline in Patients with Multiple Injuries

P. Sefrin

Head injury is the principle single lesion among patients with multiple injuries. According to own observations 91.5% of 71 such patients resulted from severe head injuries while according to Kroupa [4], 67% of 3,000 patients revealed such trauma (although these patients had solitary lesions). Even when the serious traffic accidents are decreasing in the Federal Republic of Germany, there still remain some 30,000 to 40,000 victims per year who suffer from severe brain damage [5].

A carefully-directed therapeutic attack is important for the prevention of further brain trauma. It has to start with early intensive care prior to admission. Prophylaxis of cerebral edema belongs to the preclinical therapy, as this complication can be controlled during the further course of the illness.

In addition to an intracranial increase in the intracranial volume, cerebral edema also leads to interference with the normal functioning process and metabolism. A possible prophylaxis is the administration of high doses of dexamethasone. The use of cortisone itself can have an injurious effect on the metabolism [6].

A metabolic reaction which further intervenes in many places, regulatory and stimulating, is the sympatholytic adrenaline-neural endocrine system it is generally accepted that failure of intermediary metabolism can be traced to an increased outpouring of HGH, ACTH, glucocorticoid and catecholamines acting as a buffer against the effects of severe traums [1]. For the primary post-traumatic stage an increase in sympathetic nerve activity caused by the release of adrenaline (A) and noradrenaline (NA) is characteristic. For this reason, in addition to a number of control estimations, serumadrenaline and noradrenaline were determined in patients with multiple injuries and the effects of dexamethasone on their level was examined.

The serum noradrenaline and adrenaline levels were determined by a modified method of Passen and Peuler, carried out according to Johnson and Peuler's radioenzymatic method [8][1]. Heparinized blood samples were obtained by venipuncture and placed in a tube containing solid reduced glutathione, and the tube was then placed in ice. The plasma was quickly separated by centrifugation, decanted and frozen. When the sample was to be analyzed, it was thawed, centrifuged at 4 °C for 10 minutes at 30,000 g and the supernatant directly assayed. The method is based on the enzymatic conversion of NA and A to their derivatives in the presence of catechol-*O*-methyltransferase and C-S-adenosylmethionine as the methyldonor, with subsequent conversion of these derivatives to vanillin. A group of 33 patients

1 With the friendly support of the Pharmacology Center at the University in Frankfurt (Chairman: Prof. Dr. med. D. Palm)

Treatment of Cerebral Edema
Edited by A. Hartmann and M. Brock

with head and other injuries (Group I), which were treated for 8 days with dexamethasone in decreasing doses from 8 mg to 4 mg four hourly was compared with a group of ten patients with the same injuries (Group II), who had already been given 100 mg of dexamethasone by an emergency doctor at the scene of the accident and then received for the following three days 8 mg every two hours. Thereafter, these patients received decreasing doses.
Blood samples had already been taken at the scene of the accident and were again taken after the first, second, seventh, twelfth, twenty-fourth and thirty-sixth hour. The last blood sample was taken on the fifth day after the injury.
Statistical evaluation of the data was performed with the helpful assistance of the Computer Center of the University of Würzburg and included test of standards and significance with the assistance of T- and U-tests as well as the Chi-Square test.

Results

Adrenaline and noradrenaline were increased to a maximum directly after the trauma (Figs. 1, 2). This serum-level remained constant during the first hour after the accident. Thereafter it continuously decreased over a period of five days (the total period of the experiment). No differences could be found in the *sympathetic nervous* activity which as a result of hypovolemia and hypoxia would have been shown by the release of the neural transmitter's terminal reticulum to the nerve plexuses of the pre- and post-capillary blood vessels, and the *sympathetic-adrenal* activity (which results in the simultaneous secretion of the hormones adrenaline and noradrenaline from the adrenal medulla).

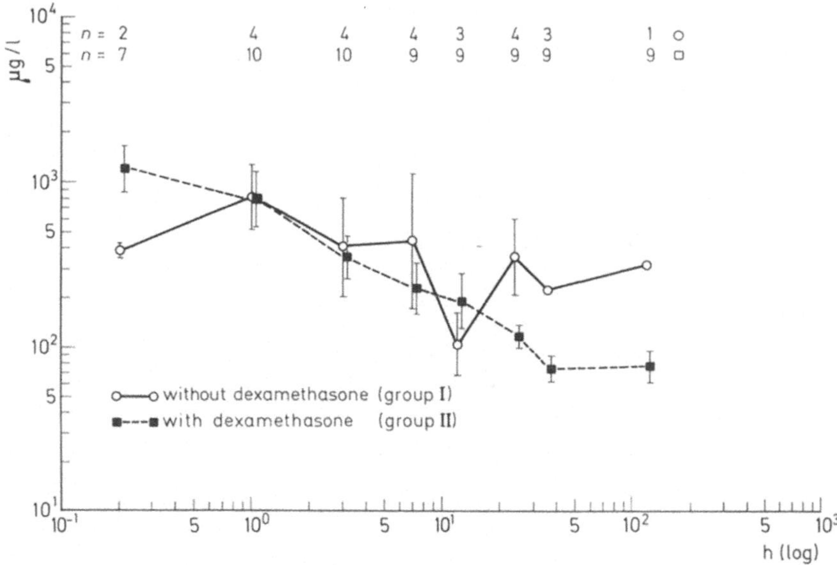

Fig. 1. Level of adrenaline in serum of patients with multiple injuries group I – without Dexamethasone, empty circles; group II – with Dexamethasone, dosage see text

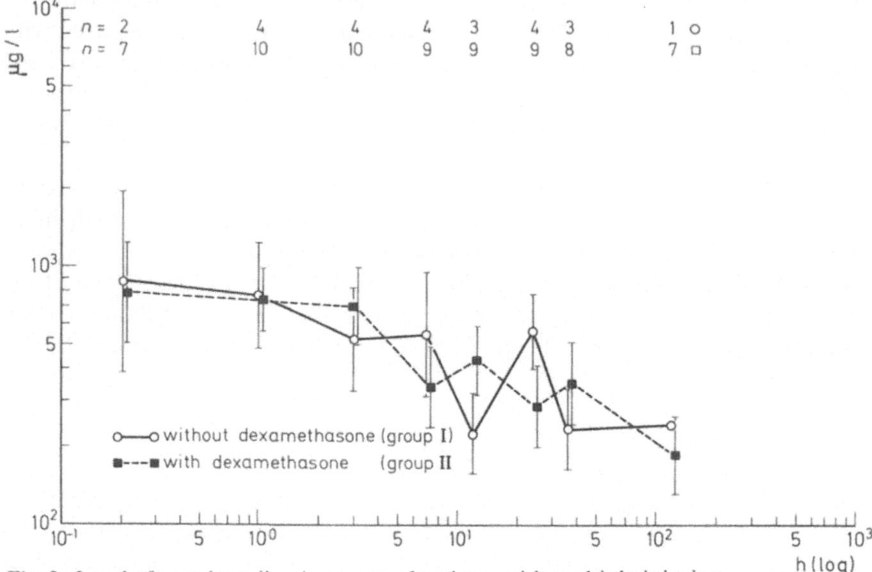

Fig. 2. Level of noradrenaline in serum of patients with multiple injuries

While the adrenaline level of Group II, which received dexamethasone at the scene of the accident, continuously decreased back to normal starting at the 36th hour, the serum level of Group I, which was not treated, remained increased in the late post-traumatic stage. One cannot come to any general, valid conclusion from this observation, mainly due to the small number of case studies in Group I. For this reason, no statistically positive significance was found (Fig. 1).

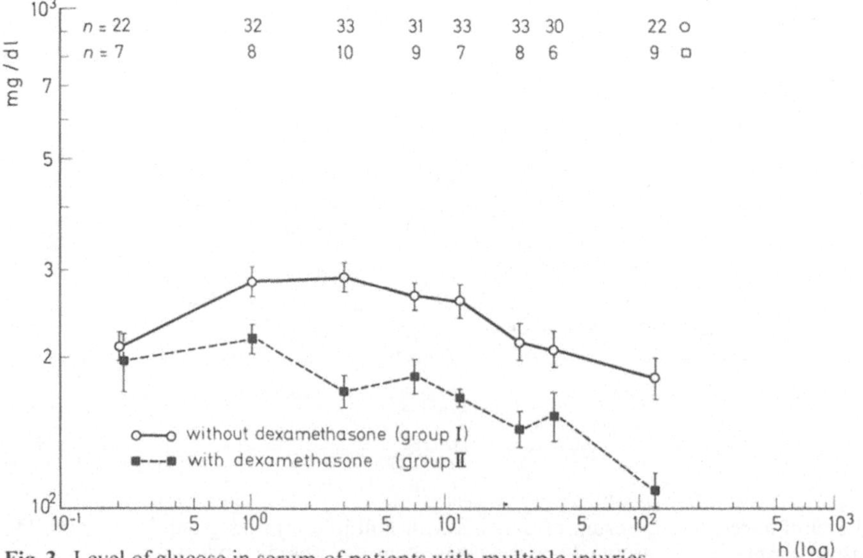

Fig. 3. Level of glucose in serum of patients with multiple injuries

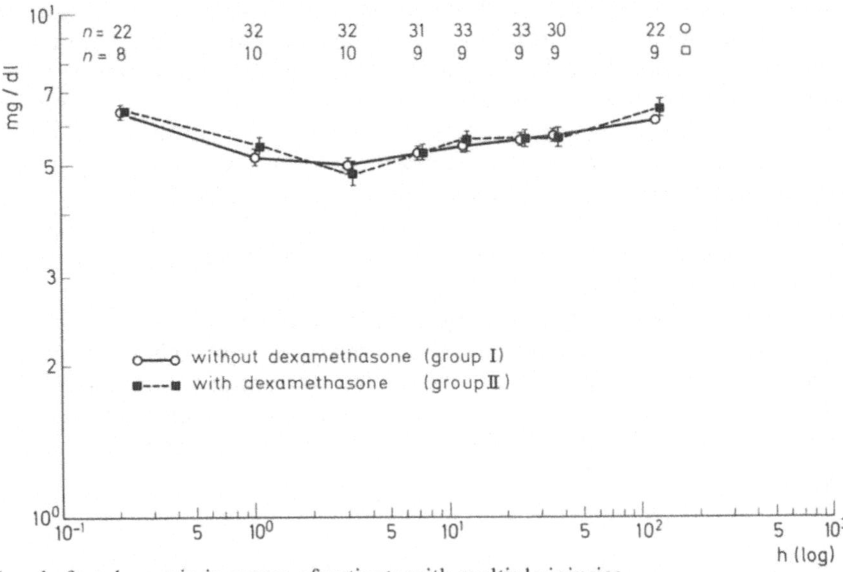

Fig. 4. Level of total-protein in serum of patients with multiple injuries

An identical curve for noradrenaline can be traced in both groups within the first few hours following the trauma (Fig. 2). From the blood samples, which followed, no significant differences were detected. As far as the level of noradrenaline is concerned, no difference can be found (Fig. 2).

Due to the influence of the glucocorticoid-level on glucose turnover (resulting in a rise of bloodsugar and reduction of glucose tolerance), on carbohydrate and protein

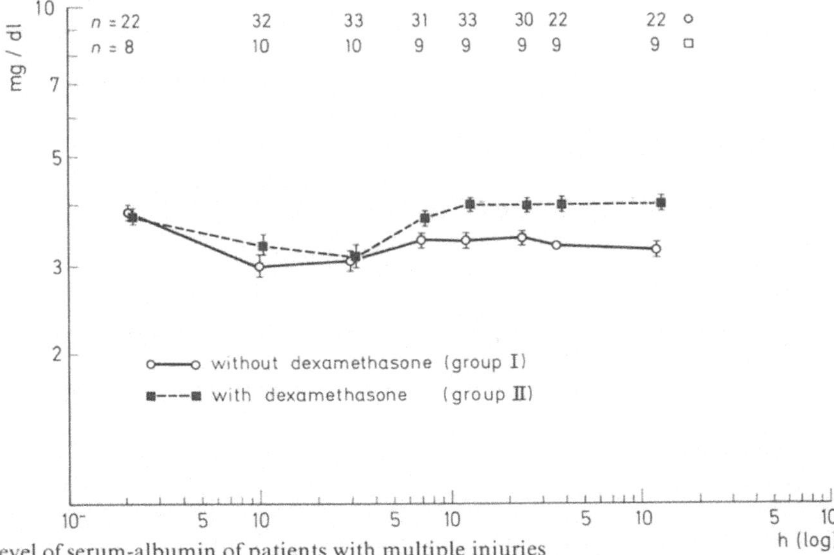

Fig. 5. Level of serum-albumin of patients with multiple injuries

metabolism, the serum glucose level, protein and albumin levels were also determined. In addition steroids produce a retention of sodium and excretion of potassium thus interfering with the electrolytes. It is obvious that the level of glucose in the serum is significantly reduced in Group II in contrast to the untreated group (Fig. 3).
A stimulation of gluconeogenesis to protect the increased energy output leads to an intensive reduction of protein. All types of protein and albumin show a distinct falling trend within the first few hours after the trauma. The increased concentration of glucocorticoid resulting from the administration of dexamethasone at the scene of the accident has no influence on this protein reduction (Fig. 4).
Within the first three hours a decrease in the albumin serum concentration can also be detected showing no differences between the two groups. Then, however, there is an enormous uptrend in group II, which leads to normal values and remains constant. In just the opposite manner, the albumin level remains statistically significantly lowered for Group I. So far so explanation can be given for these findings (Fig. 5).

Discussion

Steroids lead to an increase in reabsorption of sodium and water. Potassium is displaced from the intracellular to the extracellular compartments. In both groups, however, identical curves can be recognized in the normal range (Fig. 6). The small deviations in the median data of the serum-potassium level in the late post-traumatic stage are also within the normal range and therefore are of no value from the therapeutic point of view. Figure 7 indicates that there is also no difference in the levels of sodium between the two groups.

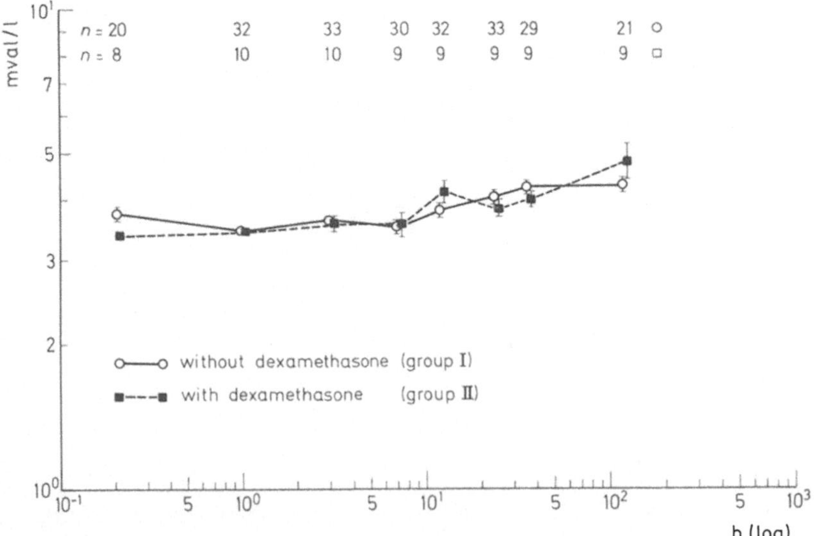

Fig. 6. Level of serum-potassium (Kalium) of patients with multiple injuries

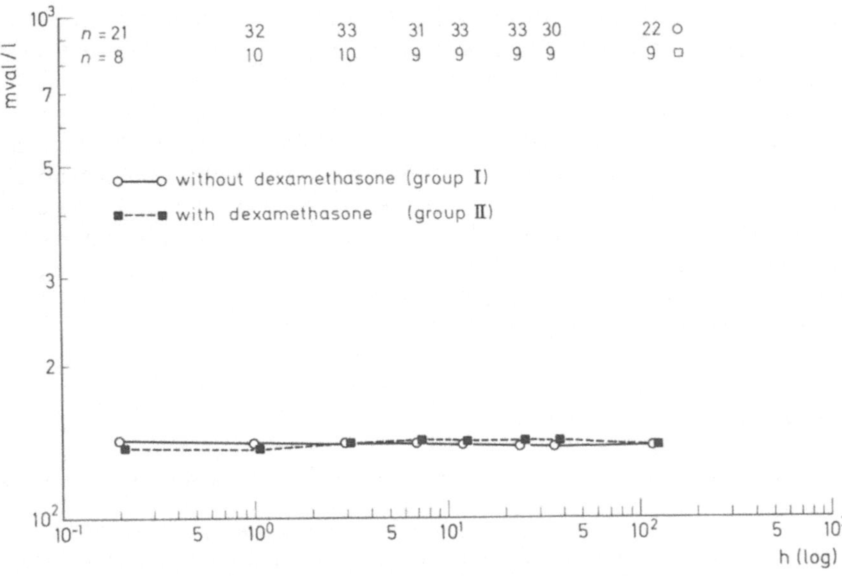

Fig. 7. Level of serum sodium (Natrium) of patients with multiple injuries

Catecholamines affect metabolism in the following sense:

1. a disturbance in glucose utilization resulting in hyperglycemia,
2. an increase of lipolysis with the increase of released fatty acids,
3. an increase of proteolysis with hypoproteinemia and a decrease of the functional proteins.

The action of catecholamines in the liver results in an increased release of glucose over glucogenolysis and gluconeogenesis. A resulting hyperglycemia is reinforced by a decrease in glucose clearance. Experiments carried out by Port and his assistants [7] indicate that infusion of adrenaline alone leads to hyperglycemia. Such a correlation cannot be found for noradrenaline. The secretion of adrenaline originates in the of the adrenal medulla in contrast to the immediate reaction of noradrenaline.

The effect of steroid on carbohydrate metabolism expresses itself in the same manner in a gluconeogenesis out of proteins and in a reduction of glucose utilization in the periphery, which leads to hyperglycemia and an increase in the consumption of protein.

Exactly the opposite reaction appeared in the patients of Group II. The significantly low glucose level can be attributed, however, to an infusion regime, where the patients were not treated with glucose during the post-traumatic stage since they suffered from a pre-existing hyperglycemia as in Group I. Undoubtfully the alteration of the findings is due to an additional stimulation of gluconeogenesis through the steroid which was administered (Fig. 3).

Dexamethasone given in high dosage at the site of the accident did not have a detrimental effect on the overall metabolism of the patients with multiple injuries.

The results agree with those of Gobiet [3], who could find no effects on the electrolyte and glucose consumption with the use of dexamethasone. However, in earlier investigations his first doses were only 24 or 48 mg and thus only one half or one fourth of the initial doses, which were given to our patients. Brandt et al. [2] have shown that in patients with severe head injuries treated with dexamethasone (2×8 mg/die) no essential impairment of the hypothalamus-hypophyseal system (controlled by LH-, FSH- and GH-secretion) could be detected. Neither the neural endocrine system nor the remaining intermediary metabolism was separately affected by the use of dexamethasone. The detectable changes are, as the comparison with identical patients from a larger research group proves, attributable to the results of the overall trauma which can be summarized by the term "injurious illness" [8]. As a result of the research done, no statements can be made concerning any definite effects on pre-existing cerebral edema.

References

1. Beisbarth H, Horatz K, Pittmayer P (1973) Bausteine der parenteralen Ernährung. Enke, Stuttgart
2. Brandt M, Wagner H, Walter W (1977) Wachstumshormon LH und FSH unter funktionsdynamischen Bedingungen im Serum sowie basale Kortisol- und Festosteron-Serumspiegel bei Schädelhirnverletzten unter Dexamethasonbehandlung. Neurochirurgia 20, 79–83
3. Gobiet W (1976) Die Behandlung eines akuten traumatischen Hirnödems. Notfallmedizin 2, 98–103
4. Kroupa J (1972) Problematik der Mehrfachverletzungen mit Beteiligung der Extremitäten. Act Chir 7, 351
5. Kunze ST (1981) Schädel-Hirn-Trauma-Editorial. Klinikarzt 10, 11
6. Labhart A (1971) Klinik der Inneren Sekretion. 2. Aufl. Springer, Berlin Heidelberg New York, p 313
7. Porte D, Grabek AL, Kuzuya T, Williams RH (1966) The effect of epinephrine on immunoreactive insulin levels in man. J Clin Invest 45, 228
8. Sefrin P (1981) Polytrauma und Stoffwechsel. Springer, Berlin Heidelberg New York

The Influence of Dexamethasone on the Midbrain Syndrome After Severe Head Injury

G. Faupel

Introduction

Previous research [1, 2, 3, 4, 5, 10] has indicated that

- early administration of high doses of dexamethasone reduces mortality [8] and has a favorable influence on the quality of survival of severely head injured patients;
- among other things, however, a larger number of stabilized unconsciously patients resulted.

Careful evaluation of all results revealed moreover that administration of high doses of dexamethasone might be associated with:

1. a lower mortality in all age groups with early administration, though naturally this includes the more severely injured patients (as, in general, they are admitted earlier),
2. lower mortality in multiple-injury cases,
3. improvement of individual neurological progress and even of all individual neurological signs, increase of vital complications not exceeding 6–8%, and in part even a reduction,
4. reduction of all classical causes of death (midbrain syndrome, secondary intracranial hemorrhage, severe wound infection, pulmonary, cardiac),
5. reduced time of confinement to bed,
6. longer survival even of those who finally die.

The present trial aimed to study cases of midbrain syndrome (MBS) and its prognosis. Since patients with midbrain damage have poorer neurological improvement and higher mortality than patients without (initial) midbrain syndrome, the possible effect of dexamethasone in these cases might be of interest.

The clinically relevant question is whether an initial or primarily existant midbrain syndrome – indicated by unilaterally or bilaterally dilated pupils, decerebrate rigidity, coma – can be influenced by steroid administration.

Patients and Methods

Except for patients in terminal stage, with open head and missile injuries, depressed fractures, or children, all critically ill patients admitted to the hospital [4] after a severe closed head injury, were included in the study. Immediately after the initial neurological examination the patients received dexamethasone or placebo accord-

Treatment of Cerebral Edema
Edited by A. Hartmann and M. Brock

ing to a continous random number. The drugs were supplied in identical appearing vials, which contained the same volume of a clear solution. Thus, physicians and nursing staff were unaware of the material being used. Group I received placebo. Group II received dexamethasone: a loading dose of 12 mg i.v. followed by 4 mg every 6 hours for eight days i.m., tapered off by daily reduction of 4 mg. Group III received dexamethasone with a loading dose 100 mg i.v. and after 6 hours again 100 mg i.m., followed as described for group II. Medical care, clots and focal mass evacuation as well as nursing, ventilation etc were provided in the same way for all patients in an intensive care unit. It should be stressed that the "placebo group" received the routine intensive care as developed during the past ten years, except for dexamethasone. Patients were examined neurologically and scored on admission and, by the same neurosurgeon, on day 3, 7, 11 using a patient evaluation sheet [6]. A final examination was performed on discharge and the results were transformed to a disability status scale [9]. The optimal total neurological score is 45 points and

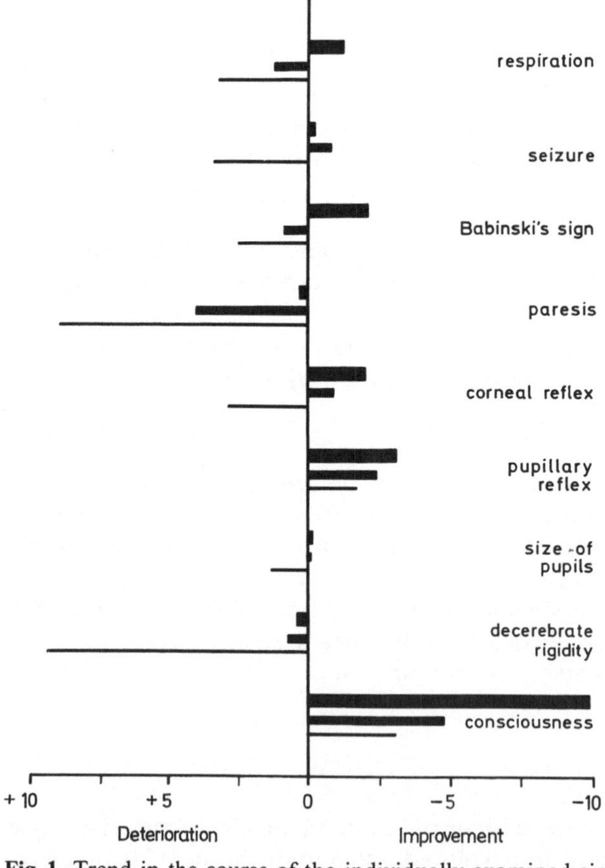

Fig. 1. Trend in the course of the individually examined signs, drawn from the difference of the mean values of days 1 and 11. Slim, mean and broad columns represent placebo, low and high dose dexamethasone respectively

274 points with brain death. There remained 95 patients in the study, 73 men and 22 women. For statistical comparison the chi-square test was used.
If we consider the individual neurological signs on the day of our examination (Fig. 1), clinical progress may be best measured on the basis of the difference of mean values from the sum of the respective scores of each therapeutic group on days 1 and 11 of our examination.

Results and Comments

It can be established that without exception all symptoms, although to varying degrees, improved under dexamethasone. A relative, although sometimes rather discrete, improvement can even be demonstrated between placebo and the low dexamethasone dosage, from days 1 to 11. There is also a positive difference in the effect between low and high dexamethasone dosage.
The greatest difference between placebo and high-dosed dexamethasone is shown with decerebrate rigidity, followed closely by paresis. There is a somewhat weaker effect on consciousness, followed by the corneal reflex and Babinski's sign. With these preconditions respiration, and more clearly convulsive seizures could be expected to have an even smaller prognostic value for the course of edema under dexamethasone treatment. At the end of this scale size of pupils and pupillary reflex would be placed, because they show the smallest difference in the neurological evaluation, to the same extent in both placebo and high dose group.
The classification according to angiographic findings (Table 1), i.e. midline displacement with or without depression of the posterior cerebral artery demonstrates that in the placebo cases, five out of seven patients die, whereas in the high dose dexamethasone group out of four patients there were no deaths. Cerebral angiography was carried out immediately after admission in 71 of 95 patients. On the basis of their angiographic results these patients were classified into three groups: in the first grade neither the anterior cerebral artery nor the posterior cerebral artery showed any displacement; in the second grade midline displacements of the anterior cerebral artery up to 30 mm were measured; patients with a midline displace-

Table 1. Angiographic findings and mortality. (Mortality in parentheses)

	Placebo	Dexamethasone		Total
		Low dose	High dose	
Cerebral anterior + posterior artery not dislocated	5 (2)	4 (1)	6 (3)	15
Midline displacement (up to 30 mm)	12 (7)	15 (4)	10 (3)	37
Midline displacement + depression of arteria cerebri posterior	7 (5)[a]	8 (4)[a]	4 (0)[a]	19
	24	27	20	71

[a] Almost $p < 5\%$

Table 2. Main causes of death in the individual treatment groups. Total sum higher than 16+10+6=32 deaths, as in two cases a clearly predominant cause of death could not be ascertained

	Main causes of death	Placebo	Dexamethasone			Total
			Low dose	High dose	Pooled	
Cerebral	Secondary MBS	7= 44%	6= 55%	1= 14%	7= 39%	14= 41%
	Primary MBS	4= 25%	2= 18%	2= 29%	4= 21%	8= 23%
	Postoperation bleeding	0	1= 9%	0	1= 6%	1= 3%
	Severe infection	0	0	1= 14%	1= 6%	1= 3%
Non-cerebral	Pulmonary	3= 19%	1= 9%	1= 14%	2= 11%	5= 15%
	Cardiac	2= 12%	1= 9%	2= 29%	3= 17%	5= 15%
	Renal	0	0	0	0	0
	Total	16=100%	11=100%	7=100%	18=100%	34=100%

ment of the anterior cerebral and a simultaneous significant depression of the proximal posterior cerebral indicating tentorial herniation, were assigned to a third degree. Although the high-dose group includes relatively fewer patients of angiographic grades 2 and 3 than the placebo group, fewer of the patients in the high-dose group died in these latter grades. This result is almost significant at the 95% level.

A further interesting point was that among the main causes of death (Table 2) in both groups the incidence of primary midbrain syndrome was approximately equal; on the other hand the incidence of secondary midbrain syndromes was higher by 30% in the placebo group (44%) than in the high-dose dexamethasone group (14%).

Above all the reduction of cerebral causes of death by treatment with high-dose dexamethasone is due to a decrease in the secondary midbrain syndrome. In the placebo group seven out of 28 patients died from brain swelling and secondary midbrain compression whereas six of 33 died in the low-dose group, and in the high dosage one out of 34. This means that secondary midbrain damage is responsible for 44, 55 and 14% of deaths, respectively.

This indicates that in the presence of tentorial herniation caused by a secondary midbrain syndrome, a reduction of mortality may be achieved by high doses of dexamethasone. The influence of dexamethasone on the primary midbrain syndrome is not so obvious, insofar as it is judged only from the small numbers involved. However, mortality of patients with midbrain syndromes was definitely lower with high-dose dexamethasone: three of 14 patients treated with dexamethasone died, compared to 11 out of 16 patients with given the placebo.

If high-dose dexamethasone can thus improve the survival rate in midbrain syndrome, the question then arises about the quality of survival.

The minimal duration of coma is nearly twice as long in cases of midbrain syndrome treated with high-dose dexamethasone than in placebo cases. Nevertheless their recovery (according to Patten et al., [9]) is not any worse, even if the cases with a 'recovery score' of '10', '9' or even '8' are substracted (Table 3).

Table 3. Out of 62 severe closed head injuries HI 30 with (primary or secondary) midbrain syndrome (MBS). Correlation between severity of head injury, duration of coma, age on the one hand and prognosis (state on discharge) on the other in midbrain syndrome (MBS) with or without dexamethasone

Out of 28 placebo 16 MBS-cases				Out of 34 high-dose dexamethasone-cases 14 MBS-cases			
Class. HI on admission (Frowein 1976)	Minimal duration of coma (days)	Age (years)	State on discharge (Patten 1972)	Class. HI on admission (Frowein 1976)	Minimal duration of coma (days)	Age (years)	State on discharge (Patten 1972)
2	2	18	1	3	6	14	5
2	4	18	10=†	2	2	64	5
3	1	17	5	3	11	18	10=†
3	6	68	10	2	4	15	6
3	4	51	10	3	11	47	8
3	5	51	10	3	11	21	9
3	6	36	6	3	11	17	10
3	11	64	10	2	11	21	9
2	1	19	5	2	2	19	5
2	11	46	10	2	11	35	9
3	1	37	5	2	11	26	10
3	5	44	10	3	11	42	9
3	3	52	10	3	11	23	9
3	8	28	10	2	10	41	8
4	3	18	10				
3	3	61	10				
2.8	4.6	39.3	8.3	2.5	8.8	28.8	8.0

Such a list can in fact clearly show that apparently many patients in the placebo group who died would have been brought to a grade of 'bare' survival quality if started with high-dose dexamethasone (score '9' or '8' according to Patten and associates, [9]). Eleven out of 16 midbrain syndrome cases in the placebo group, and ten of 14 midbrain syndrome cases in the high-dose dexamethasone group died or came to recovery scores '9' or '8', which means unconscious but stabilized or at least continuously confined to bed. These two results correlate fairly closely. Considering the other surviving midbrain syndrome cases, the final result is almost identical. One factor which may have played a role is the fact, that the high-dose cases were approximately 10 years younger.
Regarding coma, it became obvious that with one exception out of all patients with initial midbrain syndrome only those have a good prognosis (reaching a recovering degree of '6' and better in conformity with Patten et al., [9]), in whom unconsciousness does not last longer than five to six days. If the duration of coma goes beyond this point the patients die or have a very poor prognosis, with or without dexamethasone.

This highlights a very important result which is known by clinical experience but which has scarcely been verified by hard figures:
- patients with initial midbrain syndrome have primarily a worse prognosis compared to patients without;
- if the duration of coma is longer than five to six days adequate recovery cannot be expected despite dexamethasone therapy.

Table 4 reveals that in the placebo and high-dose steroid group patients with a midbrain syndrome have a less favorable neurological progress and a higher mortality than patients without an initial midbrain syndrome. After high steroid dosage, however, the two groups (with and without midbrain syndrome) show an almost equal improvement in their condition.
The table further indicates that patients with a midbrain syndrome at the time of admission generally have a qualitatively worse final outcome. None of these pa-

Table 4. Influence of initial midbrain syndrome (MBS) on final outcome and mortality. For definition of the five categories of disability see Faupel, Reulen, Müller and Schürmann 1978. (Mortality percent in brackets)

		Categories of disability					Total	
		1	2	3	4	5		
Placebo –	no MBS	0	5	1	1	5	12 (42%)	– (57%)
	MBS	1	3	1	0	11	16 (69%)	
High dose –	no MBS	5	4	3	5	3	20 (15%)	– (18%)
	MBS	0	3	1	7	3	14 (21%)	
							95 (34%)	(34%)

Examination, Admission and 1st injection (hours after accident)	1 - 2	2 - 3	3 - 6	6 - 12	12 - 24	>24
"A_1" = consciousness						
"A_2-A_4" = clouding of consciousness	○	○□	○			
"A_2-A_4" + anisocoria and / or paresis	●		■	□	○	□□
"B" = unconsciousness	○	○○	○□		○	○
"B" + anisocoria and / or paresis	○●	○	○○□	○○○■	○○ □□□	●
"B" + cerebral fits						
"B" + decerebrate rigidity	○■	○□	■■■■	○●● □■		□
"B" + muscular hypotonia = B_3				■		
"B" + respiratory disorders + pupillary reflex present	○○●	○■	■	○■	○■	○■
"B" + mydriasis + bilat. absence of pupillary reflex	■		■			
"B" + bilat. mydriasis + central apnea						
State on discharge of ○	9 5	5		9	7	9

○ high dose survived □ placebo survived ● high dose dead ■ placebo dead

Fig. 2. Correlation between depth of coma and prognosis in severely head injured patients with and without dexamethasone (details see text)

tients achieved complete recovery. Furthermore, these patients formed a large proportion of those who remained severely damaged and unconscious but stabilized. Figure 2 includes all patients of the placebo and of the high-dose steroid group. The ordinate shows the increasing deterioration of the neurological state relative to admission and the abscissa represents the interval between accident and admission or first dexamethasone injection respectively. The diagram comprises furthermore, under the marked border-line, those combinations of signs which according to the experience of Frowein [7] are associated with only the least likelihood of survival. Likewise from our own study all patients in the placebo group corresponding to a state under this border-line, died (8 patients). Contrarily in the high dose dexamethasone group six out of seven patients survived: two of those three patients who received dexamethasone early (within the first six hours) attained a final state which can be classified as having a slight to severe neurological deficit; of the patients with delayed dexamethasone treatment two patients remained apallic, a third one reached a final state of severe neurological deficit.

These findings show that with high-dose dexamethasone treatment some patients survived who otherwise might have died.

It is very likely that with early administration of dexamethasone continued on a high-dose level (100 mg initially i.v., followed by 8 mg i.v. at 2-hourly intervals) over five to seven days, as unconsciousness persists (then tapered in three days), a further improvement may be achieved, for instance by preventing a secondary midbrain compression. Of course all the other possibilities of neurosurgical intensive therapy should also be utilized namely, hyperventilation, osmotherapy, intracranial pressure monitoring, possibly the injection of corticosteroids with a more rapid onset of action, to mention but a few.

References

1. Faupel G, Reulen HJ, Müller D, Schürmann K (1976) Double-blind study on the effects of steroids on severe closed head injury. In: Pappius HM, Feindel W (eds) Dynamics of brain edema. Springer, Berlin Heidelberg New York
2. Faupel G, Reulen HJ, Müller D, Schürmann K (1977) Clinical double-blind study on the effects of dexamethasone on severe closed head injuries. In: Wüllenweber R, Brock M, Hamer J, Klinger M, Spoerri O (eds) Advances in Neurosurgery, vol 4. Springer, Berlin Heidelberg New York
3. Faupel G, Reulen HJ, Müller D, Schürmann K (1978) Dexamethason bei schweren Schädel-Hirn-Traumen. Akt traumatol 8, 265–281
4. Faupel G, Reulen HJ, Müller D, Schürmann K (1979) Dexamethasone in severe head injuries. Neurosurg Rev 2, 105–111
5. Faupel G, Reulen HJ, Müller D, Schürmann K (1980) Erfahrungen und Vorschläge zur Früh-Prognose gedeckter Schädel-Hirn-Verletzungen, insbesondere traumatischer intrakranieller Hämatome. Nervenarzt 51, 91–95
6. Faupel G, Reulen HJ, Schürmann K, Frowein RA, Penzholz H, Bushe K-A, Hübner B (1977) Begleitblatt und Verlaufskontrolle für Schädel-Hirn-Verletzte, 7. Aufl. Sharp und Dohme, München
7. Frowein RA, Steinmann HW, auf der Haar K, Terhaag D, Karimi'nejad A (1978) Limits to classification and prognosis of severe head injury. In: Frowein RA, Wilcke O, Karimi'nejad A, Brock M, Klinger M (eds) Advances in Neurosurgery, vol 5. Springer, Berlin Heidelberg New York
8. Gobiet W (1976) Die Behandlung des akuten traumatischen Hirnödems. Notfallmed 2, 98–103
9. Patten BM, Mendel J, Braun B, Curtin W, Carter S (1972) Double-blind study on the effects of dexamethasone on acute stroke. In: Reulen HJ, Schürmann K (eds) Steroids and brain edema. Springer, Berlin Heidelberg New York
10. Reulen HJ, Faupel G (1980) Behandlung des traumatischen Hirnödems mit hochdosiertem Dexamethason. In: Wieck HH (ed) Neurotraumatologie. Derzeitige Schwerpunkte. Thieme, Stuttgart New York

Clinical Use of Steroids in Cerebral Abscesses

Th. Wallenfang, H. J. Reulen, and K. Schürmann

A Historical Retrospect

Walter Dandy's [5] statement that "brain abscesses are the most vicious lesions in the brain without any question" is as true today as it was 35 years ago. Despite all the advances in diagnosis and therapy, brain abscess remains a neurosurgical challenge. Even though in the last 20 years the mortality of intracranial space-occupying processes, and especially of tumors, has been gradually brought down by advances in diagnosis and therapy and by the further development of surgical techniques, the mortality rate due to brain abscesses is still horrifyingly high. According to comprehensive clinical surveys, it is between 30 and 45% [4, 9, 16, 20, 27]. In the case of multiple cerebral abscesses and of abscesses localized especially in the midbrain, the pons, the cerebellum, and in the ventricle region, the prognosis is still less favorable. Practically all the authors report that when the brain abscesses occur in these localizations, the course is as a rule fatal [6, 10].

The introduction of antibiotics into the therapy of cerebral abscess was undoubtedly able to reduce the mortality rate from more than 60%–40% [4, 6], but chemotherapy did not fulfill other expectations associated with it. Our own investigations, and those of other authors [9, 10, 16] in recent times, reveal that since the introduction of antibiotics there has been no further essential reduction in the mortality rate. This lack of improvement cannot be attributed to any change in the etiology or in the pathogen spectrum, which is in agreement with the literature [9, 10, 26]. The rhinogenic and otogenic route is still the commonest portal of entry of the pathogenic organisms. Staphylococci and streptococci are standing at the top of the pathogenic spectrum.

The high mortality rate caused by the disease is still ascribed, inter alia, to the persistent difficulties with the diagnosis of cerebral abscess, due to the nonspecificity of the associated symptoms. The result is that treatment is delayed [4, 10, 26]. The diagnostic difficulties are also reflected in the high mortality. Thus, where the diagnosis had been certain or suspected, the mortality rate among our patients was 30%, while when the space-occupying lesions were of uncertain origin or the diagnosis had been incorrect this figure rose to 50%; this clinical experience is in agreement with observations reported by other authors [4, 9]. In many cases the concomitant inflammatory symptoms were actually obscured by the antibiotic treatment, making the diagnosis still more difficult.

Axial computed tomography currently ensures an early diagnosis in a high proportion of the cases, an exact localization of the lesion, and information on its size, the associated edema, and any capsule formation [14, 28]. What is of particular val-

Treatment of Cerebral Edema
Edited by A. Hartmann and M. Brock

ue is the differentiation between multilocular abscesses, subsidiary abscesses ("daughter" abscesses) in the direct vicinity of the cerebral abscess, and multiple abscesses, as well as the possibility of following the further course, whether postoperatively or in exclusively conservative treatment. The faster diagnosis made possible by this method of examination and the associated timely start of treatment make a further reduction of the mortality seem likely.

A further reason given for the lack of an improvement in the clinical results in addition to the delay in starting treatment is inadequate administration of antibiotics, inadequate both as regards the dose and the choice of the antibiotic itself [10, 26]. Apart from this, there is still no unanimous agreement on the timing and type of the surgical intervention [4, 9, 10, 27]. Mortality rates ranging between 10 and 50% have been given by different authors for the particular surgical techniques (aspiration, drainage, excision) [8, 13, 17].

A critical evaluation of the literature shows that the composition of the patient material is very diverse, the most important factors for the outcome of the disease, namely the patient's state of consciousness and the stage of the abscess, whether acute or chronic, are only rarely taken into consideration. The overall impression is that each surgical technique results in particularly high mortality when it is carried out in the acute inflammatory stage of an abscess while the necrotizing process is still going on and when the state of consciousness is deteriorating.

A cerebral abscess is an infectious, intracranial, space-occupying lesion. By giving the patient effective antibiotic treatment the infectious side of the inflammatory process can be brought under control, but not the space-occupying aspect caused by the inflammatory edema. Therefore, the results will not be improved until effective measures are taken against the cerebral edema in the acute stage together with the antibiotic therapy, and currently steroids appear to be the best answer to the problem. Although many authors attribute the high mortality rate primarily to irreversible damage to the midbrain caused by cerebral edema and the raised intracranial pressure, steroids have not become established as a form of treatment and their use is still disputed [10, 23, 25].

In 1978 Garfield [10] complained of the lack of any clinical work on the efficacy of steroids in cerebral abscess, but at the same time he warned of the danger of reducing the immunological defences if steroids were used in inflammatory brain diseases. Likewise, there was still no suitable experimental work on animals that would permit a systematic investigation of acute and chronic brain abscesses and of the changes in inflammatory cerebral edema.

The aims of the present study are to draw attention to the need for improvement in the state of consciousness pre-operatively and, by means of effective conservative treatment, to bring the abscess to a state optimal for its surgical removal.

According to the analysis of our clinical material we are justified in hoping that, by using the correct strategy of treatment, we can reduce the mortality of cerebral abscess decisively insofar as the various factors affecting the prognosis are taken into account. On the basis of results from the animal experiments it should be possible to consolidate our clinical experience.

Clinical Material

The clinical study is based on 110 brain-abscess patients who had been admitted between 1958 and 1980. The brain abscess was acute in 36 of the patients and chronic in 74. In 91 cases the clinical findings were confirmed at operation and by the histological and microbiological investigations. Nineteen patients were treated exclusively by conservative measures. There were 94 solitary abscesses in the cerebral hemispheres, six solitary abscesses affected more than one lobe, one solitary abscess was close to the ventricle, three were in the cerebellum, and two in the pons. Ten patients had multiple brain abscesses.

No significant change in the etiology could be established over the 22-year period in question. Hematogenous metastatic cases [36], rhinogenic or otogenic ones [29], and post-traumatic cases [28] were of practically equal significance.

Among the pathogens detectable in abscess puncture samples from only 40 of our patients staphylococci occurred most frequently (40%), followed by streptococci (20%). In the majority of cases no pathogenic organisms could be cultured from the abscess material, owing to the preceding antibiotic treatment.

Between 1958 and 1973 53 brain-abscess patients were treated exclusively with antibiotics. The mortality in this group was 41%. It is not just the high mortality rate under exclusive antibiotic treatment that demonstrates its limitations. In spite of the great progress made in the development of antibiotics, the incidence of brain abscess has not decreased. Among the 110 patients seen in the 22 years, 45 cases were diagnosed in the last five years.

Since 1972, in addition to the treatment with antibiotics dexamethasone has been given to 53 patients in doses of 4×4 mg to 4×8 mg/day. The treatment was started on the day of admission and continued until the 6th to 8th day after the operation. In exclusively conservative treatment, and especially in the case of multiple abscesses, the duration of the steroid treatment is governed by the progress of the edema in the computer tomograms.

Prognostic Factors

Now that modern antibiotic therapy has made it possible to control the infectious aspect of cerebral abscess, clinical experience shows that the persistently high mortality is due largely to the concomitant inflammatory brain edema, the raised intracranial pressure, and secondary damage to the midbrain structures. These factors determine the consciousness level of the patient (grade I–IV), which must be regarded as the most decisive prognostic factor. Among our 110 patients the mortality increased in proportion to the increasing impairment of consciousness. Thus, the mortality was 13% in patients who had arrived at the clinic in a fully alert state, 33% in drowsy patients, 59% in stuporose patients, and 80% in patients admitted in a state of coma.

The second important factor determining the prognosis is the type of the abscess, i.e. whether the latter is acute or chronic. The mortality in patients with an acute brain abscess was distinctly higher than in patients with a chronic abscess, at all four levels of consciousness (Fig. 1).

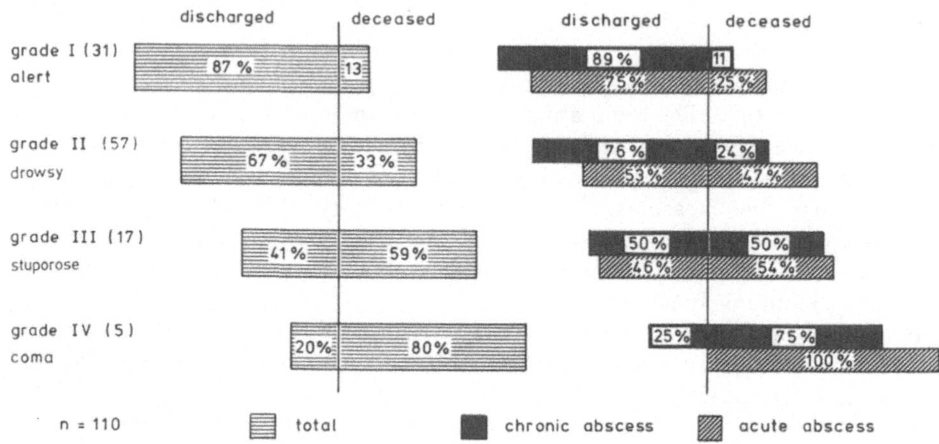

Fig. 1. Relationship between the state of consciousness (grade I–IV) on admission to hospital and the mortality in patients with acute and chronic brain abscess

Even in the fully alert patients (grade I) the mortality for the acute abscess was about twice as high (25%) as in the patients with chronic brain abscess. If both factors together are taken into consideration to evaluate the patient's chances, the prognosis was most unfavorable in those in a stuporose and comatose state and suffering from an acute abscess, while fully alert patients with a chronic abscess have the best chances of survival.

The third important prognostic factor is the site of the abscess. Abscesses situated in the midbrain or multiple abscesses had a definitely less favorable prognosis than solitary hemisphere abscesses.

Among our 10 cases of multiple brain abscesses too the (3) patients survived only when a state of full consciousness or drowsiness could be reached and where the multiple abscesses had been situated exclusively in the cerebral hemispheres.

Since the two prognostic factors that can be influenced, the pre-operative level of consciousness and the type of the abscess, play a decisive part, a clear reduction in the mortality rate should be achievable by controlling the infectious cerebral edema and by converting the inflammatory process from acute into chronic.

Clinical Results

Comparison of two similar groups of patients with and without steroid treatment thus allows one to decide to what extent steroids can improve the individual level of consciousness by reducing cerebral edema.

In the group of patients treated with dexamethasone in addition to the antibiotics there were 18 fully alert patients, in whom no deterioration set in. In the patients with some impairment of the level of consciousness an improvement was found in all stages, and especially in the patients who were drowsy.

Of the 19 patients drowsy on admission, improvement to a fully conscious state proved possible in 15 cases. None of the patients deteriorated. Among the 13 stupo-

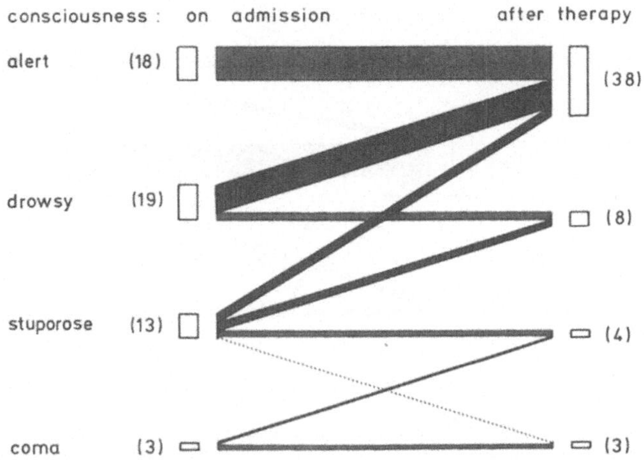

Fig. 2. The alterations in the state of consciousness under treatment with antibiotics in combination with steroids. 47% of the patients show an improvement and only 2% show a deterioration of consciousness

rose patients five improved to a state of clear and four to a state of impaired consciousness, three patients remained stuporose. Only one patient (with multiple abscesses) deteriorated. Of the five patients with multiple brain abscesses treated with steroids, three improved and survived (Fig. 2).

In comparison with this, only a few patients improved when antibiotics were given on their own, three drowsy and three stuporose patients progressing to the next better state of consciousness. Of the 11 conscious patients, ten remained at the same level (grade I), while one deteriorated. In the state of drowsiness (grade II), 17 patients showed no alterations but ten deteriorated; three stuporose patients (grade III) remained at the same level of consciousness and one deteriorated. The patients who had been admitted in deep coma (grade IV), and in many cases already with neurological signs of midbrain compression, had a poor prognosis both with or without the steroid treatment (Fig. 3).

If we summarize the individual results for the various levels of consciousness, an essentially more favorable picture is found for the group treated with steroids in combination with antibiotics. The patient's level of consciousness improved in 47% of the cases, remained unchanged in 51%, and deteriorated in only 2%. When antibiotics were given on their own, on the other hand, an improvement in the level of consciousness could be achieved in only 13% of the cases, remaining unchanged in 66% and deteriorating in 23%.

The surgical procedure has also changed since the introduction of steroids. Whereas before 1972 the surgical intervention, whether aspiration or excision, was carried out shortly after admission, under antibiotic protection, nowadays in the majority of the cases the inflammatory brain edema can be controlled by dexamethasone. In this way there is sufficient time for antibiotic treatment before the operation and for the limitation of the local inflammatory process that it brings about. If a progressive improvement occurs in the level of consciousness, one can safely wait until the optimum time for excision arrives.

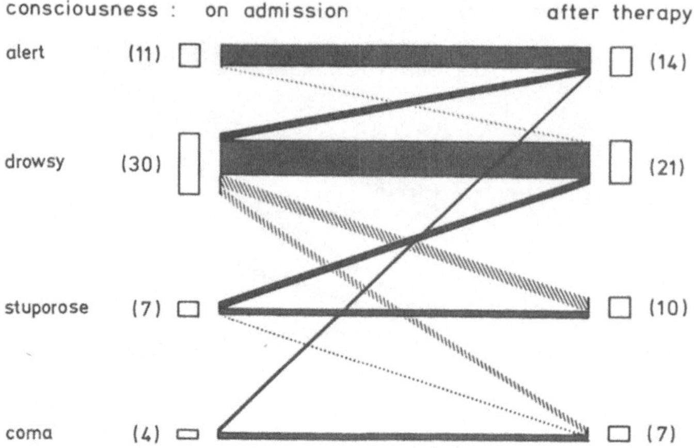

Fig. 3. The alterations in the state of consciousness under treatment with antibiotics alone. Without steroids only 13% of the patients show an improvement but 23% show a deterioration of consciousness

The usefulness of this preliminary treatment with a combination of antibiotics and steroids is also evident from the operation results. When the operation was carried out after the combined therapy it was possible to reduce the acute abscess mortality to 47% and the chronic abscess mortality to 10%. When the operation was performed under antibiotic protection alone the results were essentially less favorable, the mortality being 89% for the acute abscesses and 30% for the chronic abscesses.

This could give the impression that the low surgical mortality in the group of patients treated with dexamethasone should be attributed to the improved level of consciousness pre-operatively. However, it was found that, for the same level of consciousness and the same surgical technique, the mortality after the combined treatment was always lower, a point that deserves special emphasis.

The patients with multiple abscesses and abscesses localized centrally in the basal ganglia, in whom no operation was possible, showed a substantially more favorable course with the combined treatment.

Whereas in the pre-steroid era all the patients with multiple abscesses (five cases) had died, 50% of such cases (six patients) survived when dexamethasone had produced a reduction of the brain edema before secondary midbrain and brainstem damage led very quickly to coma and death.

The improved chances of survival in patients with supratentorial multiple abscesses with additional steroid therapy is clearly demonstrated by the following case.

A 12-year-old boy with multiple abscesses was stuporose on admission and the CT-scans over a period of three months served as a guide in the follow-up of the brain inflammation. Under the combined therapy with dexamethasone and antibiotics the

→

Fig. 4. 12-year-old patient with multiple brain abscesses, admitted to hospital in a drowsy state of consciousness. Under the antibiotherapy in combination with dexamethasone, there was a rapid neurological improvement. One aspiration of the encapsulated abscess in the right temporoparietal lobe was performed and the patient was discharged in a good state of health

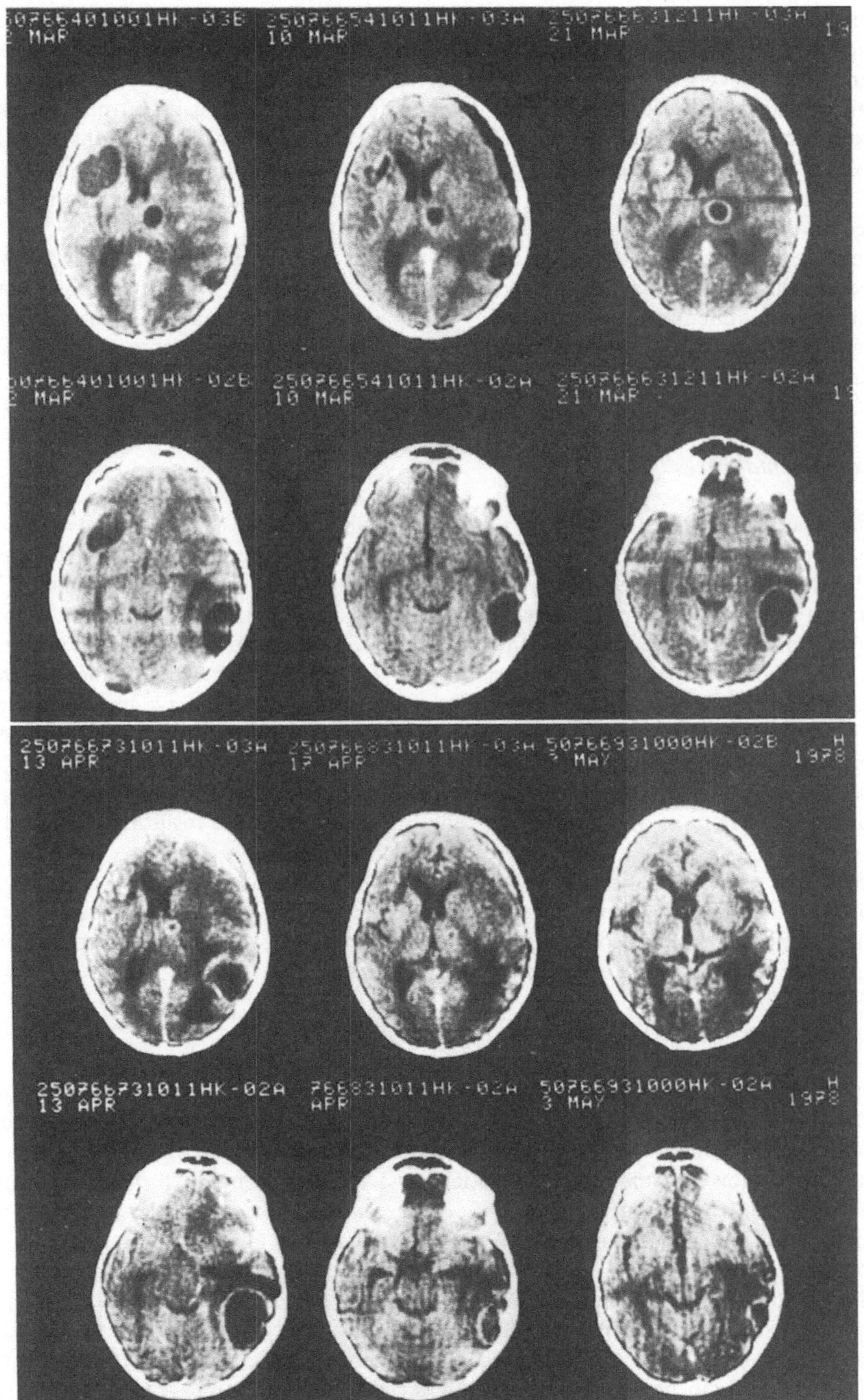

10 MAR
21 MAR
10 MAR
21 MAR
13 APR
17 APR
1978
250766731011HK-02A
13 APR
3 MAY
1978

clinical condition of the patient improved. In addition there was a uniform reduction of the edema and the space-occupying effect, and the ring enhancement became progressively more uniform. Corticosteroids were discontinued twice, and the patient's state of consciousness then deteriorated and he had a grand mal attack, though the CT showed no increase of ring enhancement. After three months of high doses of antibiotics, in addition to a reduced dose of dexamethasone and a puncture of the abscess in the right parietal lobe in the chronic state, the boy was discharged free from symptoms (Fig. 4).

Antibiotics obviously remain the basis of the treatment of cerebral abscess. However, in the light of our clinical investigations we have been able to establish that antibiotic treatment on its own is often incapable of preventing a deleterious outcome in states of acute inflammation, because of the very acute manner in which the edema sometimes develops.

Experimental Investigation

Our experimental investigation into artificial brain abscesses in cats emphasizes the necessity for the addition of steroids into the treatment of brain abscess, and the usefulness of dexamethasone in the management of inflammatory cerebral edema.

Brain abscesses were produced by the stereotactic inoculation of an agar-bouillon culture of Staphylococcus aureus, the most common organism in our clinical investigations. Treatment was then started on the seventh day, by which time the inflammatory brain edema had reached its maximum and the intraventricular pressure was nearly eight times as high (22.6 ± 4.0 mm Hg) as in the control group receiving only a sterile agar-bouillon mixture. In this state of increased intracranial pressure due to the acute brain abscess and its edema, the animals were in great danger on account of the herniation of the brain stem and the resulting changes in the midbrain.

Treatment with antibiotics alone (50 mg cefazedone/kg/day) and in combination with dexamethasone (50 mg cefazedone/kg/day and 0.5 mg dexamethasone/kg/day), given over a period of either three or thirteen days, was compared, special attention being given to the effect of the steroid:

1. on the clinical picture,
2. on the appearance of the CT,
3. on the water content in the white matter surrounding the abscess.

Under the combined treatment with antibiotics and dexamethasone the clinical state of the animals improved markedly within the first three days. Whereas the state of consciousness often improved even after 24 h, the anisocoria and the paresis exhibited a slower remission. Antibiotic therapy on its own still produced no appreciable neurological improvement after three days. A decrease of the symptoms of raised intracranial pressure was only observed as the antibiotic treatment progressed.

The CT follow-up studies on the seventh day showed extensive edema around the area of tissue necrosis, with a shift of the ventricular system to the left. The extravasated contrast medium increased, depending on the extent of the disturbance of the blood-brain barrier, and the irregular ring enhancement reached its maxi-

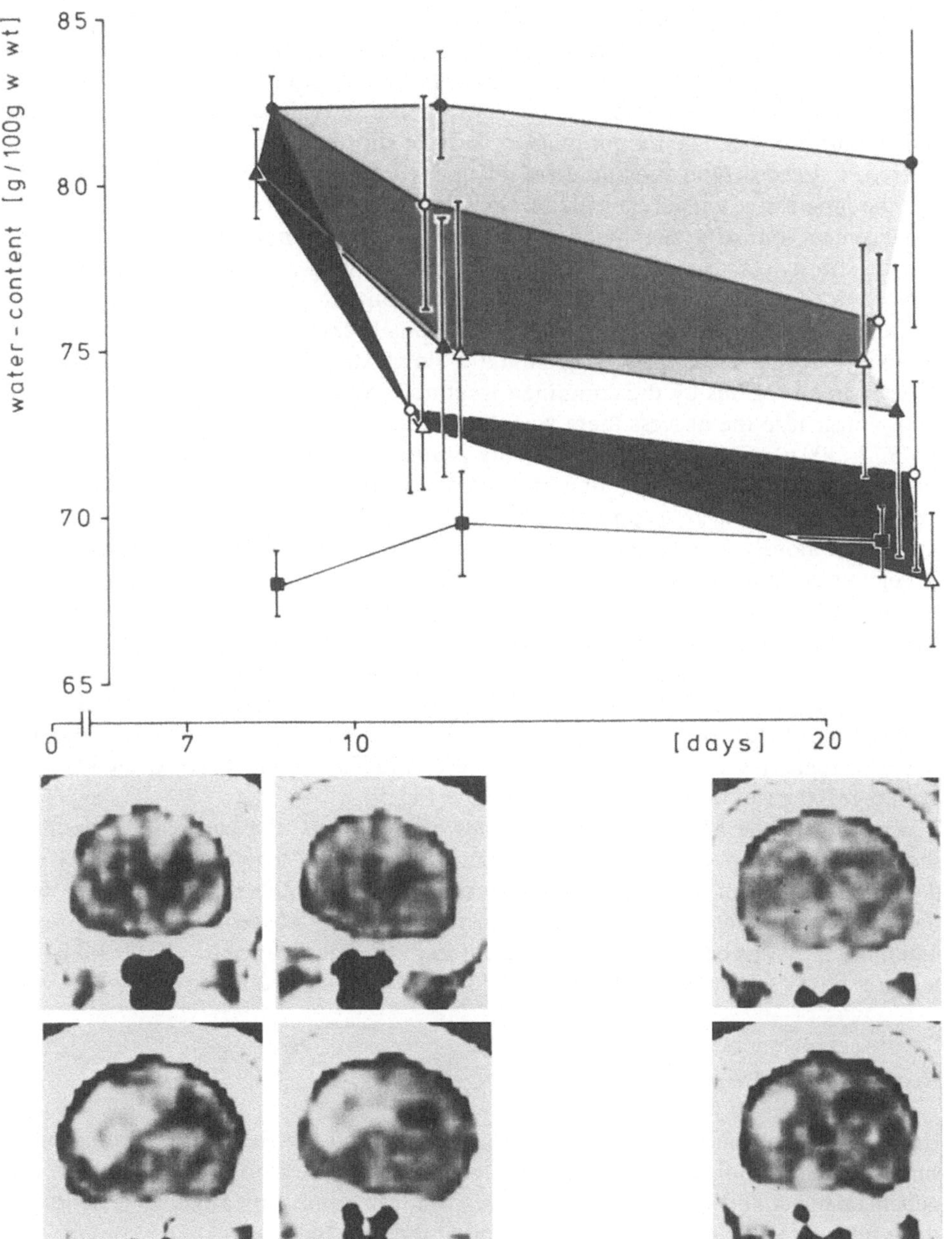

Fig. 5. Changes of water content (g/100 g wet weight) of the white matter adjacent (circle), remote (triangle) and contralateral (square) to the abscess. Therapy was started when the edema reached its maximum (7th day after Staphylococcus aureus inoculation). Black area antibiotics in combination with steroids, dark grey area antibiotics alone, light grey area without any therapy. Mean and standard deviation are given. The CT-scans correspond to the water content of the different days under therapy with antibiotics and steroids (first line without contrast medium, second line 10 min after contrast injection). Note the correlation between decreasing water content and the improving blood brain barrier

mum 10 minutes after the injection of the contrast medium. The animals that did not improve with medical treatment all showed an increase in the size of the abscess as well as an increase in the intensity of the ring enhancement. However, when the antibiotic treatment was combined with dexamethasone, the space-occupying effect and the surrounding edema diminished and the shift of the ventricular system decreased. In accord with the stabilization of the compromised blood-brain barrier and the progressive capsule formation, on the tenth day there was a decreased ring enhancement soon after the injection of the contrast medium (Fig. 5).

The superiority of the combined treatment over that with antibiotics alone is clearly demonstrated by the measurements of the water content.

While the water contents in tissue adjacent to the abscess were high in the untreated group (7th day 82.3 g/100 g wet weight, 20th day 80.0 g/100 g), they were markedly reduced in all regions by the combined treatment within the first three days. In regions adjacent to the abscess there was a reduction of 11% (83.2 g/100 g wet weight to 73.2 g/100 g). Further reduction of the brain edema was minimal in the immediate vicinity of the abscess, but progressed to normal values (68.0 g/100 g wet weight) in the remote areas up to the 20th day.

Antibiotics alone produced no statistically significant reduction of the brain edema in regions close to the abscess in the first three days. The water content was only slightly reduced, from 82.3 g/100 g wet weight on the seventh day to 79.4 g/100 g on the tenth day. After 13 days of antibiotics only the cerebral edema was still very marked in the immediate vicinity of the abscess on the 20th day, as shown by the water content (75.8 g/100 g wet weight). In regions remote from the abscess, on the other hand, the water content fell in the first three days of the treatment, but then remained in the pathological range, as in the regions close to the abscess, at 74.6 g/100 g wet weight until the 20th day (Fig. 5).

If we compare the action of the two types of treatment, the combined treatment shows a distinct superiority over antibiotics on their own, which is particularly evident in alterations of the water content in regions close to the abscess. The substantially lower water content in the area surrounding the abscess under the combination therapy was confirmed in a multiple test at a significance level of $\alpha = 0.01$ after three days of therapy (tenth day) and 13 days of therapy (20th day).

Risk of Steroid Therapy

However, in the combatting of the cerebral edema and the rise of intracranial pressure by the administration of dexamethasone the question arises whether the beneficial effect of the steroids may not be counterbalanced by an adverse action of these substances, i.e. delayed encapsulation of the abscess.

Among our patients who were given adequate antibiotic treatment no activation of the cerebral infection was ever observed.

However, the indiscriminate use of steroids in abscess therapy is not without risk, especially when the patient has been admitted in a disturbed state of consciousness and the diagnosis is still unclear. While a CT-scan showing a lesion with ring enhancement and surrounding edema is characteristic of an abscess, gliomas and metastases may also show similar features.

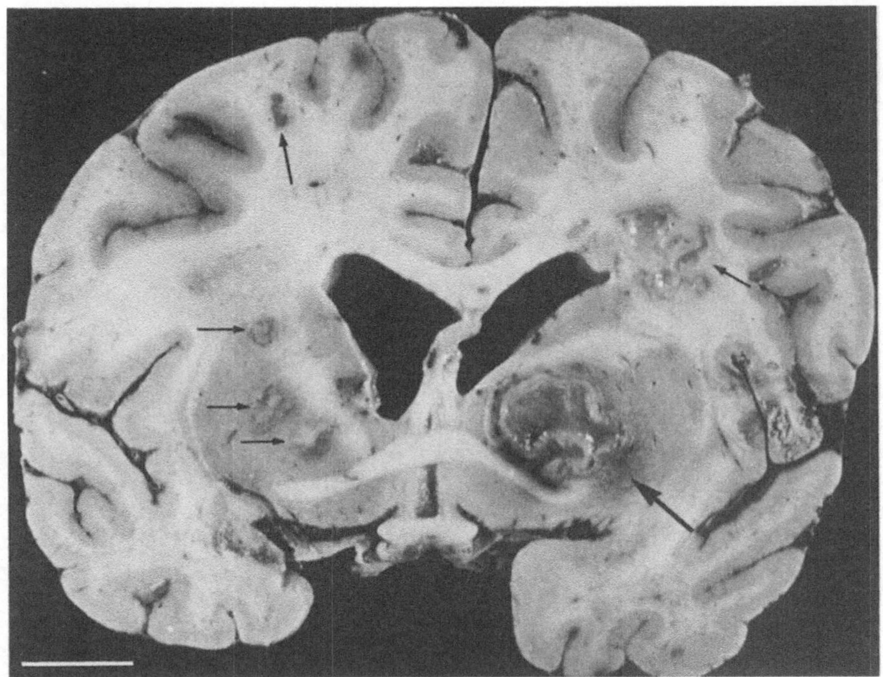

Fig. 6. Multiple intracerebral abscesses (most of them are acute → some are older ➞ with obvious capsule formation) in the brain of a 73-year-old woman who developed 24 days before death a slowly progressive cerebral coma. During the last ten days she was treated with corticosteroids alone, as she was thought to have a brain tumor. (Fixation in an aqueous solution of formaldehyde; frontal sections; scale bar 2 cm)

Three patients with brain abscesses treated exclusively with dexamethasone after an erroneous diagnosis of glioblastoma died in a very short time. All had shown a brief improvement in the state of consciousness at the start of the treatment.

In two cases autopsy revealed that activation of a chronic brain abscess had occurred as a result of the anti-inflammatory effect of the steroid (Fig. 6). Besides the chronic brain abscess, multiple acute abscesses were found after therapy with dexamethasone alone. Around the acute brain tissue necrosis there was only a slight proliferation of the blood vessels and only a slight inflammatory and mesenchymal reaction (Fig. 7).

The animal studies confirmed impressively the experiences obtained in the clinical field. Administration of glucocorticosteroids on their own in an inflammatory cerebral abscess has disastrous results. Extensive and virtually areactive zones of necrosis developed around the abscess, with no reduction of the disturbance of the blood-brain barrier; in particular the fibrinoid vascular wall necroses were surrounded by a fibrin-rich exudate without any appreciable inflammatory reaction.

These possibly adverse effects of steroids on the mesenchymal and glial reaction desired in cerebral abscess have not been observed in our experimental studies after three days of the combined treatment. However, they did become manifest, after 13-days of combined antibiotic and steroid therapy, as a delayed formation and insufficient strength of the abscess capsule.

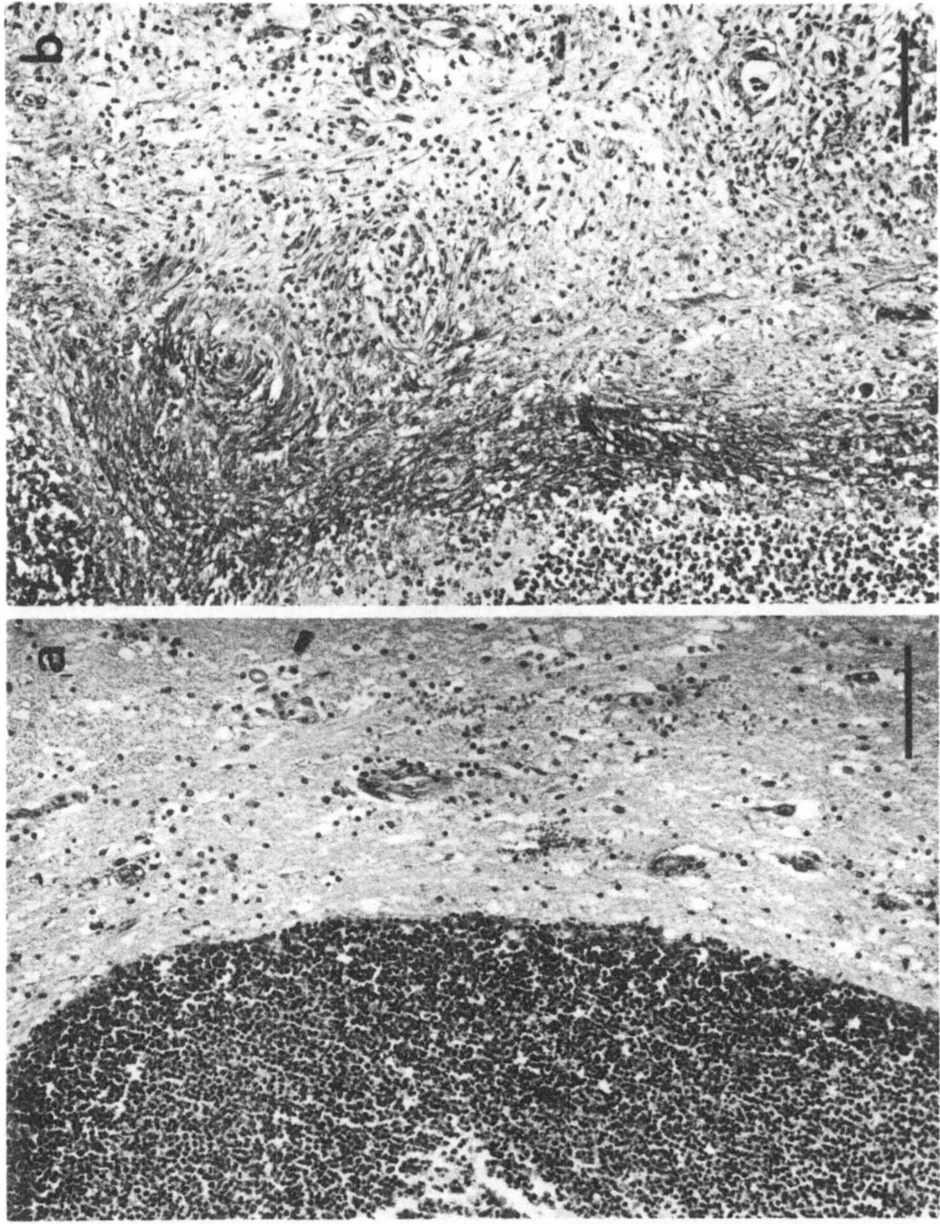

Fig. 7a, b. Intracerebral abscesses in a 73-year-old woman treated with corticosteroids only. **a** Acute abscess in the white matter. Note the distinct border of the inflammatory brain defect with absence of any cellular, vascular or glial reaction in the neighborhood. **b** Chronic abscess with formation of a thick capsule with mesenchymal, glial and inflammatory elements (older than 10 days). (Same magnification as in **a**.) (Paraffin embedding; HE; scale bar 0.1 mm)

Discussion

Analysis of the data on 110 patients with cerebral abscesses shows that the prognosis is already largely established on admission by the extent of the raised intracranial pressure, the cerebral edema, and the midbrain compression on the one hand and by the activity of the infection on the other hand. Thus, the prognosis was most favorable in fully conscious patients suffering from a chronic cerebral abscess, very poor in stuporose and comatose patients with acute abscess, and practically hopeless in patients with multiple brain abscesses.

This immediately shows the need for early diagnosis and exact localization, both of which are currently made possible by computed tomography. Any delay in diagnosis, especially in the case of an acute lesion, can thwart all subsequent therapeutic measures by a fulminating development of inflammatory cerebral edema and elevation of the intracranial pressure. Thus, in our patients we found that even adequate antibiotic treatment, often prior to the establishment of the diagnosis, must be regarded as inadequate treatment. This was shown by the deterioration of the conscious level in 23% of the cases and the absence of neurological improvement in 66%, so that any surgical intervention was also associated with a high risk. In many cases the patients' progressive clinical deterioration actually caused frequent changes of antibiotics and their combinations, mistakes that have also been described by other authors [9].

The persistently poor prognosis under antibiotic therapy on its own demonstrates that the infectious process is not alone in determining the prognosis; another factor is the course of the concomitant cerebral edema. Maxwell [19] and Ransohoff [24] were the first to report good experiences with the treatment of cerebral edema in brain abscess.

The action of dexamethasone therapy consists in an effective control of the cerebral edema and of the raised intracranial pressure, as a result of which the state of consciousness improved in 47% of the patients. Even stuporose and comatose patients with multiple brain abscesses, who previously nearly always died when treated with antibiotics only, frequently displayed a neurological improvement under the steroid therapy. Finally, a deterioration of the state of consciousness was only observed in 2% of the cases under the additional steroid therapy.

Analysis of our investigations shows that by using the combined antibiotic and dexamethasone treatment valuable time is gained for the antibiotic treatment, thanks to the improvement in the pre-operative level of consciousness. The time gained and also the control of the infectious lesion increase the chances of an encapsulation of the abscess, which represents a further prognostic improvement since it is thus possible to convert an acute, local, inflammatory lesion into a chronic and locally circumscribed one. Under these favorable preconditions excision of the abscess represents the best surgical measure, and in individual cases the mortality can be reduced to 10%.

Our experiences of intracerebral abscess in the experimental animal [30] also demonstrate that the additional treatment with dexamethasone together with an antibiotic leads to a significant reduction of perifocal inflammatory edema, which results in a marked improvement of the clinical course.

After only three days of antibiotic treatment in combination with dexamethasone, practically equal water contents within the normal range were achieved in the regions both close to and remote from the abscess, whereas antibiotic treatment on its own still had not eliminated pathologically high water contents even after 13 days of treatment.

The striking neurological improvement of the animals under the additional dexamethasone treatment certainly cannot be attributed solely to the rapid reduction of the brain edema in the first three days, as is also suggested by the studies of other authors [1, 11, 12, 21, 22]. Besides the mechanical action as a cement-substance between the broken cells of the blood-brain barrier, the steroids exert a regulating effect by modifying the cell metabolism [18]. In earlier studies we were able to show that with the steroid treatment, faster repair processes take place in the blood-brain barrier and the risk of hypoxemic damage to the cells can be reduced [3]. However, an essential prerequisite for any steroid action is still the structural integrity of the edematous tissue [29], which makes it necessary to limit the spread of the inflammatory necrosis as quickly as possible, by appropriate antibiotic treatment.

The studies by Kazner et al. [15] give a general picture of the different kinds of ring formation in the computer tomogram due to the variety of the pathological conditions. Our own computer-tomographic studies under standardized experimental conditions revealed the development of the abscess and the extent of the perifocal disturbance of the blood-brain barrier. The changes in the edema and kinetics of the injected contrast medium permitted statements to be made about the stage of the abscess.

When the blood-brain barrier was disturbed in the acute state of inflammation, the irregular ring enhancement after the injection of a contrast medium was present mainly as an extravascular iodine component and reached its maximum extent ten to twenty min later. When the blood-brain barrier was restored (repaired) three days after treatment with antibiotics and dexamethasone, we were able to observe a marked reduction of the brain edema around the abscess, a return to normal of the displaced ventricular system, and a ring structure with maximum enhancement soon after contrast injection, which must be attributed to predominant intravascular distribution of the contrast medium.

For the clinical practice this means that ring enhancement in the CT cannot be simply equated with abscess capsule formation. This is in accord with the results of Enzmann et al. [7] who demonstrated in abscess studies on dogs, that the ring structure seen in the earliest stage is identical with the zone of inflammation. Therefore, the age and the evolution of the abscess cannot be determined on the basis of a single CT-investigation. The state of consciousness, the laboratory data, and the altered dynamics of the inflammatory process in a sequence of CT scan determine the timing and the nature of each surgical procedure.

The advantages of dexamethasone should not allow us to forget the risks associated with all steroid therapy. The weakening of the immunological defences and the anti-inflammatory action of steroids are precisely the reasons quoted as objections to dexamethasone treatment in cerebral abscess [10, 23]. Although in our patient material no activation of the cerebral infection was observed, in patients treated with dexamethasone and antibiotics a risk of delayed capsule formation still exists when the steroid is given in excessive doses or for too long a time. Histopathological investigations in animals with brain abscess treated with antibiotics and dexamethasone for 13 days showed a delayed development and a lack of firmness of the capsule [2]. As the edema had regressed almost completely after only three days of dexamethasone treatment, and suppression of the glial and mesenchymal reactions must be regarded as slight at this time, it is recommended to start with high doses of dexamethasone under antibiotic protection and to reduce the steroids to a minimum as the neurological improvement continues. On the other hand, the antibiotic treatment should be continued for at least four to six weeks, since up to this time we were able to detect by electron microscopy pathogens capable of division in the abscess material, whereas the microbiological investigations gave negative results at an earlier stage.

Although the use of dexamethasone in addition to antibiotics has proved to be advantageous for controlling the inflammatory brain edema and gaining time for capsule formation, it is dangerous to administer steroids alone, especially in patients with a disturbed state of consciousness and when the diagnosis has not been confirmed. As both clinical experience and experimental results have shown, a brain abscess treated exclusively with dexamethasone develops widespread tissue necrosis with little or no inflammatory reaction but with marked damage to the blood-brain barrier on account of the progressive toxic effect of the bacteria.

Treatment with antibiotics in combination with steroids represents the most reliable method for patients with disturbances of consciousness both as regards the neurological improvement and the elimination of the inflammatory focus; in our experience it promises the best prospects of ultimate recovery in the pre-operative and post-operative stages.

Summary

It is an established fact that patients with a brain abscess are at very great risk. Rapid and reliable diagnosis by computed tomography and the further development of effective antibiotics have certainly contributed to a reduction of the mortality rate due to this disease, but an essential reduction to below 40% has not yet been achieved in spite of all the advances.

On the basis of the results obtained in a group of 110 patients we attempted to analyse the essential reasons responsible for this high mortality rate. The outcome of the disease is affected not so much by the infectious process as by the associated inflammatory cerebral edema with secondary midbrain damage. If it is impossible to bring the developing cerebral edema under control with the often very rapid progress of the raised intracranial pressure, even the best antibiotic treatment will not arrest the increasing deterioration in the level of consciousness. The prognosis is thus decisively dependent on whether the pre-operative state of consciousness can be improved and whether the abscess can be converted from the acute into the chronic stage. It is only by the use of steroids in addition to appropriate antibiotic therapy that an effective reduction of the edema can be achieved. Treatment with dexamethasone buys time, during which an abscess capsule can develop, and in addition the improved state of consciousness represents an essential prerequisite for successful surgical intervention. The fact that patients with multiple brain abscesses survive nowadays is certainly a result of steroid therapy.

Experimental studies on cats with brain abscess support the clinical findings. The rapid neurological improvement, the reduction of the edema, and the repair of the blood-brain barrier prove that combined antibiotic-steroid treatment is invariably superior to antibiotics alone.

The possible dangers of steroid therapy, such as a reduced state of defence and anti-inflammatory action, do not outweigh the enormous advantages of reducing the edema, which constitutes a completely calculated risk when the treatment is correctly applied.

References

1. Baethmann A, Oettinger W, Rothenfußer W, Kempski O, Unterberger A, Geiger R (1980) Brain edema factors: Current state with particular reference to plasma constituents and glutamate. In: Advances in Neurology 28. Cerbós-Navarro J, Ferszt R (eds). Raven Press, New York, pp 171–195
2. Bohl J, Wallenfang Th, Bothe HW, Schürmann K (1981) The effect of glucocorticoids in the combined treatment of experimental brain abscess in cats. In: Advances in Neurosurgery, vol 9. Schiefer W, Klinger M, Brock M (eds). Springer, Berlin Heidelberg New York, pp 125–133
3. Bothe HW, Wallenfang Th, Khalifa A, Schürmann K (in press) The relationship between brain edema, energy metabolism, glucose content and rCBF by artificial brain abscess in cats. In: Advances in Neurosurgery, vol 10. Driesen W, Brock M, Klinger M (eds). Springer, Berlin Heidelberg New York
4. Carey ME, Chou SN, French LA (1972) Experience with brain abscess. J Neurosurg 36:1–9
5. Dandy WE (1946) Craniotomy and total dissection as a method in the treatment of abscesses of the brain. Ann Surg 123:805–806
6. Davidoff LM (1934) How to obviate failures in the results of surgery of brain abscess. Laryngoscope (St Louis) 44:871–875
7. Enzmann DR, Britt RH, Yeager AS (1979) Experimental brain abscess evolution: computed tomographic and neuropathologic correlation. Radiology 133:113–122
8. French LA, Chou SN (1974) Treatment of brain abscess. In: Advances in Neurology, vol 6. Thompson RA, Green JR (eds). Raven Press, New York, pp 269–275
9. Garfield J (1969) Management of supratentorial intracranial abscess. A review of 200 cases. Brit Med J 2:7–11
10. Garfield J (1978) Brain abscess and focal suppurative infections. In: Vinken PJ, Bruyn GW (eds) Handbook of Clinical Neurology 33. Amsterdam New York Oxford, pp 107–147
11. Hansebout RR, Lewin MG, Pappius HM (1972) Evidence regarding the action of steroids in injured spinal cord. In: Steroids and brain edema. Reulen HJ, Schürmann K (eds). Springer, Berlin Heidelberg New York, pp 153–155
12. Herrmann HD, Neuenfeld D, Dittmann J, Paleske H (1972) The influence of dexamethasone on water content, electrolytes, blood-brain barrier and glucose metabolism in cold injury edema. In: Steroids and brain edema. Reulen HJ, Schürmann K (eds). Springer, Berlin Heidelberg New York, pp 77–85
13. Jooma OV, Pennybacker JB, Tutton GK (1951) Brain abscess: Aspiration, drainage or excision? J Neurol Neurosurg Psychiat 14:308–313
14. Kazner E, Lanksch W, Steinhoff H, Wilske J (1975) Die axiale Computer-Tomographie des Gehirnschädels. Anwendungsmöglichkeiten und klinische Egebnisse. Fortschr Neurol Psychiat 43:487–574
15. Kazner E, Steinhoff H, Wende S, Mauersberger W (1978) Ring-shaped lesions in the CT scan – differential diagnostic considerations. In: Advances in Neurosurgery, vol 6. Wüllenweber R, Wenker H, Brock M, Klinger M (eds). Springer, Berlin Heidelberg New York, pp 80–85

16. Le Beau J, Creissard P, Redondo A (1972) Sur le prognostic des abcès du cerveau. Neuro-Chirurgie 18:181–188
17. Le Beau J, Creissard P, Harispe L, Redondo A (1973) Surgical treatment of brain abscess and subdural empyema. J Neurosurg 38:198–203
18. Long DM, Maxwell RE, French LA (1972) The effects of glucosteroids upon experimental brain edema. In: Steroid and brain edema. Reulen HJ, Schürmann K (eds). Springer, Berlin Heidelberg New York, pp 65–67
19. Maxwell RE, Long DM, French LA (1972) The clinical effects of a synthetic glucocorticoid used for brain edema in the practice of neurosurgery. In: Steroids and brain edema. Reulen HJ, Schürmann K (eds). Springer, Berlin Heidelberg New York, pp 219–232
20. Morgan H, Wood MW, Murphey F (1973) Experience with 88 consecutive cases of brain abscess. J Neurosurg 38:698–704.
21. Ortega BD, Demopoulos HB, Ransohoff J (1972) Effect of antioxidants on experimental cold-induced cerebral edema. In: Steroids and brain edema. Reulen HJ, Schürmann K (eds). Springer, Berlin Heidelberg New York, pp 167–175
22. Pappius HM (1972) Effects of steroids on cold injury edema. In: Steroids and brain edema. Reulen HJ, Schürmann K (eds). Springer, Berlin Heidelberg New York
23. Quartey GRC, Johnston JA, Rozdilsky B (1976) Decadron in the treatment of cerebral abscess. An experimental study. J Neurosurg 45:301–310
24. Ransohoff J: The effects of steroids on brain edema in man. In: Steroids and brain edema. Reulen HJ, Schürmann K (eds). Springer, Berlin Heidelberg New York, pp 211–217
25. Rosenblum ML, Hoff JT, Norman D, Weinstein PR, Pitts L (1978) Decreased mortality from brain abscesses since advent of computerized tomography. J Neurosurg 49:658–668
26. Samson DS, Clark K (1973) A current review of brain abscess. Amer J of Med 54:201–210
27. Schiefer W, Klinger M (1978) Aspects of modern brain abscess. Diagnosis and treatment. Neurosurg Rev 1:37–45
28. Shaw MDM, Russel JA (1977) Value of computed tomography in the diagnosis of intracranial abscess. J Neurol Neurosurg Psychiat 40:214–220
29. Tutt HP, Pappius H (1972) Steroids and brain edema. In: Reulen HJ, Schürmann K (eds). Springer, Berlin Heidelberg New York, pp 147–155
30. Wallenfang TH, Bohl HJ, Kretzschmar K (1980) Evolution of brain abscess in cats; formation of capsule and resolution of brain edema. Neurosurg Rev 3:101–111

The Effect of High Doses of Dexamethasone on Cerebral Blood Flow in Patients with Cerebral Tumors

C. Buttinger, A. Hartmann, R. von Kummer, and J. Menzel

Accumulation of edematous fluid due to cerebral tumors leads to increase of intracranial pressure (ICP) with subsequent reduction of regional cerebral blood flow (rCBF). The value of prolonged administration of steroids to patients suffering from tumors of the brain is well known since the early reports of Ingraham et al. [4] and Tytus et al. [10]. Studies on the influence of various doses of steroids on ICP in patients with supratentorial tumors [5] and tumors of the posterior fossa [2] have indicated that ICP can be adequately lowered by dexamethasone. Own experience has indicated that cerebrospinal fluid pressure in patients suffering from supratentorial malignant brain tumors decreases more slowly than the clinical condition improves [1]. Therefore factors other than ICP alone must be influenced by the administration of dexamethasone. Since rCBF is not triggered by intracranial pressure alone we have studied this particular factor. This preliminary report presents observations on the effect of high doses of dexamethasone on rCBF in patients suffering from malignant brain tumors and proven edema.

Method

rCBF was measured by the nontraumatic method using inhalation of Xenon 133 [3, 7]. After inhalation of the gas from an 8-litre airbag desaturation curves were recorded over both aspects of the skull for ten min and stored in a desk computer. Thirty-two clearance curves were corrected for recirculation by simultaneous recording of Xenon 133 activity in the end exspired air, since this reflects the activity in the arterial blood. Alteration of the original clearance curve by contamination from extracerebral tissue was mathematically corrected by considering the tail of the curve as being influenced only by this tissue part and the so-called slowly perfused tissue (white matter). Finally the computer printed data about rCBF of the fast perfused tissue.

Since the blood-tissue partition-coefficient lambda in pathological tissue such as the tumor or the edematous part is unknown, an rCBF-parameter (ISI) was used which does not take lambda into consideration. ISI calculates rCBF from the original desaturation curve between the second and third minute [3, 9].

Our studies in patients without central nervous system diseases have revealed that ISI is ± 55 ml/100 g/min.

If necessary all data were corrected for $PaCO_2$ with a factor of 4% ISI per mm Hg $PaCO_2$ deviation.

Eleven patients entered the protocol. Diagnosis of intracerebral tumor was es-

Treatment of Cerebral Edema
Edited by A. Hartmann and M. Brock

Table 1. Patients data

No. of patients	Sex	Age	Diagnosis	Side with tumor
1	f	57	Solitary metastasis	R
2	f	67	Meningioma of the sphenoid ridge	R
3	f	71	Glioblastoma	L
4	f	70	Glioblastoma	L
5	f	60	Glioblastoma	R
6	f	45	Multiple metastases	R+L
7	f	61	Astrocytoma	L
8	f	54	Solitary metastasis	L
9	f	57	Oligodendroglioma	R
10	m	53	Solitary metastasis	R

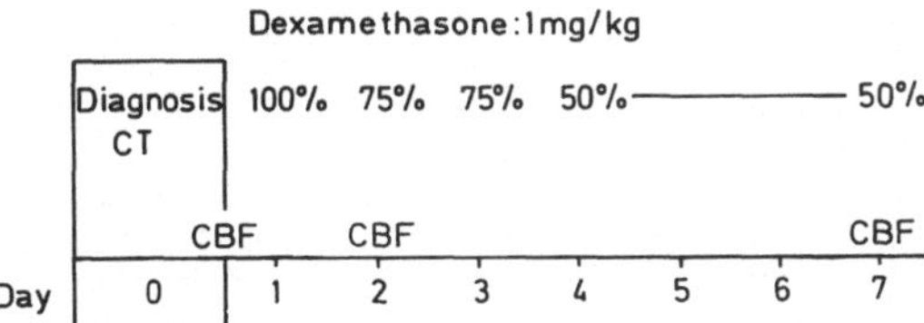

Fig. 1. Protocol of the study

tablished by clinical examination, angiography and EEG in all cases. The diagnosis and presence of brain edema with tissue shift was confirmed by cranial computer tomography in all cases. In one out of the 11 cases the final diagnosis did not show the existence of a tumor. The case was excluded from consideration. Diagnosis, age, sex and brain side of involvement are listed in Table 1. Except patient 6, who was shown to suffer from multiple metastases, all patients had their neoplasm only on one side of the brain. rCBF was measured three times, before start of dexamethasone therapy (CBF_{ss}), one day (CBF_2) and seven days (CBF_3) after the start. A high dose (1 mg/kg bodyweight) was used on the first day with subsequent reduction (Fig. 1).

Results

Table 2 indicates the mean rCBF of both hemispheres before the start of treatment and rCBF-alterations on day 1 and 7. Before the start of treatment in cases 1, 4, 8 and 9 mean rCBF of the involved side was significantly lower than in the hemisphere with no tumor. In patient 3 – who suffered from a highly vascularized glioblastoma – the rCBF on this side was higher than that of the contralateral hemisphere. In the other five cases there was no significant difference between the two sides. However, focal flow reduction in these five cases was more prominent on the side of the tumor. This means that in these five patients reduction of rCBF in the non-involved side was more generalized than in the hemisphere with the tumor, which showed the same mean rCBF but higher interregional differences.

Table 2. Mean regional cerebral blood flow (CBF_{SS}) before start of dexamethasone treatment and percentage alteration one day (CBF_2) and one week (CBF_3) after start of treatment

No. of patients	$PaCO_2$ (mmHg)	Hemisphere with tumor				Hemisphere without tumor			
		Side	CBF_{SS} (ml/100 g/min)	Difference (%) CBF_{SS}/CBF_2	Difference (%) CBF_{SS}/CBF_3	Side	CBF_{SS} (ml/100 g/min)	Difference (%) CBF_{SS}/CBF_2	Difference (%) CBF_{SS}/CBF_3
1	40	R	48.6	+10.2±21.3	+15.7±26.0	L	54.5	+ 0.5±20.9	+11.5±32.7
2	40	R	47.2	− 2.1± 9.9	+14.2±24.3	L	46.0	− 0.1±12.9	+17.7±27.6
3	36	L	49.8	+ 5.5±10.8	+ 4.9±15.8	R	40.5	+ 9.9±15.6	+12.4±17.1
4	39	L	39.8	−14.9±11.5	+25.7±22.0	R	45.9	−10.7± 9.7	+22.8±21.2
5	38	R	33.6	+10.5±13.6	+ 2.3±26.4	L	35.3	+17.8±25.9	+15.3±39.0
6[a]	41	R[a]	51.3	−10.7±24.6	− 2.1±22.0	L[a]	53.7	−13.6±18.2	+ 2.4±22.0
7	45	L	64.6	+ 3.3±14.8	+23.0±11.1	R	63.1	+ 8.7±25.4	+22.7±11.2
8	45	L	65.9	− 4.3±12.7	+ 1.3±19.8	R	74.3	− 0.4±12.8	+ 1.9±11.0
9	41	R	31.3	+12.1±14.9	+33.2± 9.9	L	36.7	+ 7.6± 6.3	+10.1±11.0
10	34	R	37.2	−13.7± 4.6	+27.4± 9.8	L	37.1	−15.1± 6.4	+14.0± 4.1

CBF_{SS} mean CBF before start of dexamethasone administration; $CBF_{2/3}$ mean CBF one/seven days after start of therapy

[a] Patient with multiple metastases in both hemispheres

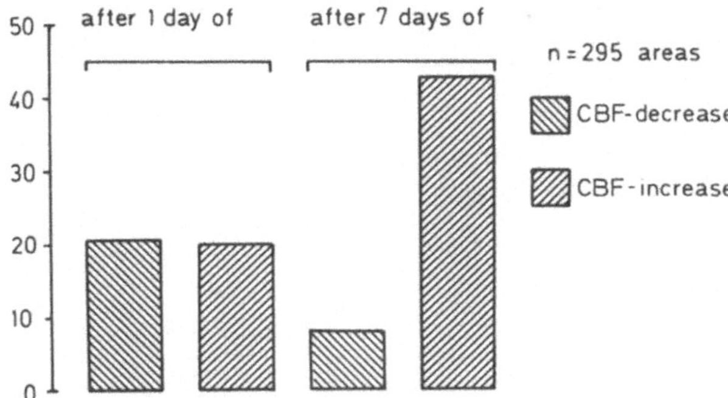

Fig. 2. Percentage of areas with significant rCBF-change during administration of dexamethasone

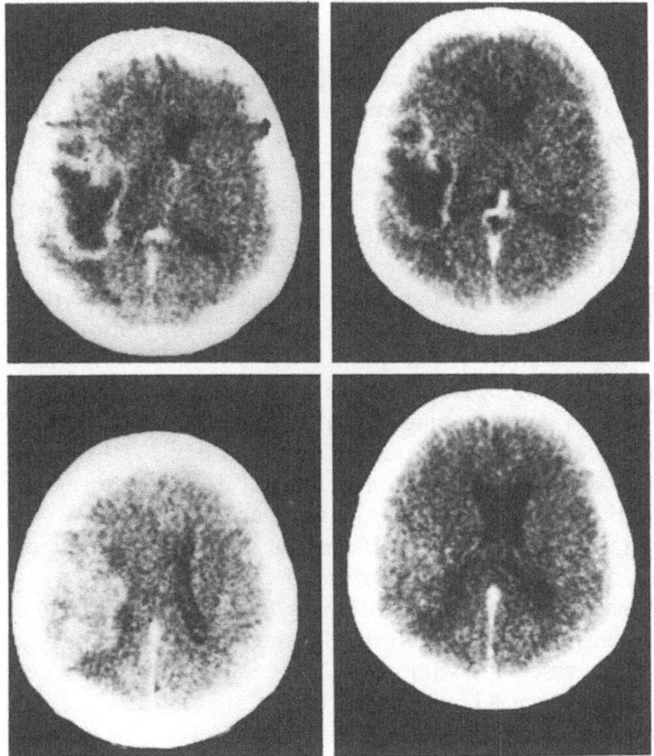

Fig. 3. Cranial computer-tomography with enhancement before (left side) and seven days after start of dexamethasone treatment. Before start of treatment there is an extensive midline shift to the right in this case with a left-sided glioblastoma. Seven days after start of dexamethasone both lateral ventricles are visible

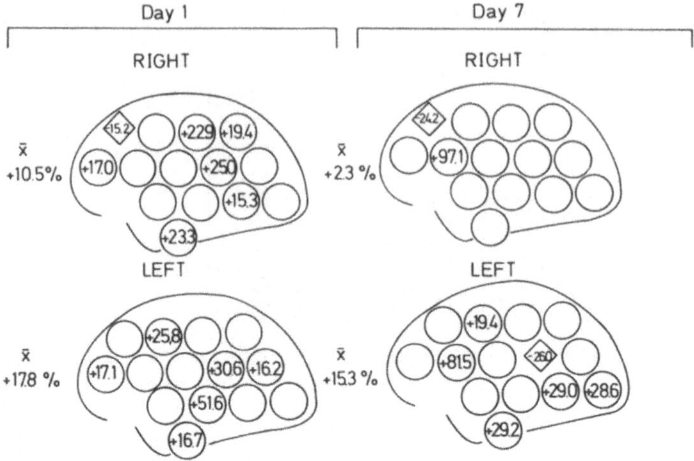

Fig. 4. rCBF-change in percentage (compared to steady state flow) one and seven days after start of dexamethasone. Filled circles indicate significant rCBF-increase, rhombs significant rCBF-reduction. The patient suffered from a right-sided tumor. rCBF-change was more prominent on the side with no tumor

After starting treatment mean rCBF did not increase significantly (more than 15%, Ref. [3]) till CBF_2 in any tumor-hemispheres but it did in one non-tumor hemisphere (case 5). In one hemisphere without neoplasm (case 10) mean rCBF decreased by more than 15%.

At time of CBF_3 the mean rCBF showed a significant increase in five out of ten tumor-hemispheres and in four out of ten hemispheres with no tumor. Only two patients presented with significant rCBF increase on both sides (patients Nr. 4 and 7). In none of the cases rCBF was there any significant drop from CBF_{ss} till CBF_3.

From these data it might be concluded that hemispheric CBF does not respond sufficiently within one day of the start of therapy but that in 50% of all cases CBF increases until day 7. This impression is supported by the regional calculation. Alteration of rCBF of more than 15% can be considered as being significant [3]. Figure 2 indicates the percentage of all 295 areas with significant rCBF-increase and -decrease on day 1 and 7, respectively. On day 1 (CBF_2) 20% showed a significant increase of flow and 20.6% a significant decrease. Seven days after start of treatment (CBF_3) only 8.1% of all calculated areas presented with significant drop of rCBF, but 43.1% showed a significant increase. This correlated well with diminution of edema as estimated from repeated CT-scans (Fig. 3).

There was no uniform pattern to show which of the hemisphere in the individual patients responded more to dexamethasone. Figure 4 for instance represents the data of case Nr. 5 with no mean change on day 1 in the tumor-side but significant CBF-change (+17.8%) on the contralateral side. Regional calculation indicated that seven areas in the involved side presented with significant rCBF-increase and one area with a significant rCBF-decrease. On day 7 again the tumor-hemisphere showed no significant mean change of flow with one focal increase and one focal decrease, whereas the tumor-free hemisphere showed a significant mean increase of rCBF, due to five areas with rCBF-elevation and one area with a drop in rCBF.

Discussion

If the ICP is increased on account of a brain tumor and subsequent edema it decreases rather slowly during dexamethasone treatment [5], whereas the level of consciousness might improve after one day of administration and even earlier if higher doses are used [1, 6]. Plateau waves which may lead to critical intracranial pressure situations diminish in duration and height within 12 hours [1]. The positive effect of dexamethasone on the appearance of plateau waves on the first day seems not to be correlated with any recognizable effect on cerebral blood flow. No significant improvement of CBF in the tumor side was observed in any of our cases. The number of areas with significant regional rCBF-improvement was identical to that with rCBF-deterioration.

After seven days of treatment hemispheric CBF was improved in nine out of 20 hemispheres (ten patients). This confirms the observations of Reulen et al., who measured significant increase of CBF in one side after 5–7 days of treatment with 24 mg dexamethasone per patient [8], and other authors [11]. The data from this study indicate that in five patients more areas showed a significant rCBF-increase than showed a significant rCBF-reduction. This focal rCBF-improvement was more prominent on the tumor side than on the contralateral one. Still, rCBF increased in both sides, thus raising the question why dexamethasone acts on the side without detectable edema in the CT-scan. It might be that the hemisphere with the neoplasm and edema compresses the contralateral side thus leading to reduced blood flow by transhemispheric ICP-increase. Furthermore, slight edema with damage to the cellular metabolism might be present but not recognizable in CT-scans. A general reduction of rCBF on both sides due to transneural depression might also be beneficially influenced by dexamethasone.

This study does not give any conclusive answer about the mode of action of dexamethasone. The effect of the steroid on rCBF was independent of the steady state value, which means that tissues both with reduced and with normal flow showed improvement of rCBF after seven days of treatment (Fig. 4). This might point to a more generalized effect. On the other hand did the tumor-hemispheres present with more areas of increased flow after therapy than the contralateral sides which might indicate that the action of dexamethasone is more specific. At present a decision cannot be made with the clinical approach used in this study. However, since rCBF – in accordance with ICP-reduction – might already be improved two days after the start of treatment, a corresponding investigation is now in progress.

References

1. Alberti E, Hartmann A, Schütz H-J, Schreckenberger F (1978) The effect of large doses of dexamethasone on the cerebrospinal fluid pressure in patients with supratentorial tumors. J Neurol 217: 173–181
2. Brock M, Zillig C, Wiegand H, Zywietz C, Mock P (1976) The effects of dexamethasone on ICP in cases of posterior fossa tumors. In: ICP III, Beks JWF, Bosch DA, Brock M (eds). Springer, Berlin Heidelberg New York, pp 236–243
3. Hartmann A, v Kummer R (in press) Die atraumatische Messung der regionalen Gehirndurchblutung: Methodik und Zuverlässigkeitsprüfung. Fortschr. Neurol.

4. Ingraham FD, Matson DD, Mc Laurin RL (1952) Cortisone and ACTH as an adjunct to the surgery of craniopharyngiomas. New Eng J Med 246:568–571
5. Kullberg G (1972) Clinical studies on the effect of corticosteroids on the ventricular pressure. In: Steroids and brain edema. Reulen H, Schürmann K (eds). Springer, Berlin Heidelberg New York, pp 253–258
6. Maxwell RE, Long MD, French LA (1972) The clinical effects of a synthetic glucocorticoid used for brain edema. In: Steroids and brain edema. Reulen H, Schürmann K (eds). Springer, Berlin Heidelberg New York, pp 219–232
7. Obrist WD, Thompson HK, Wang HS, Wilkinson WE (1975) Regional cerebral blood flow estimated by Xenon 133 inhalation. Stroke 6:245–256
8. Reulen HJ, Hadjidimos A, Schürmann K (1972) The effect of dexamethasone on water and electrolyte content and on rCBF in perifocal brain edema in man. In: Steroids and brain edema, Reulen HJ, Schürmann K (eds). Springer, Berlin Heidelberg New York, pp 239–252
9. Risberg J, Ali Z, Wilson EM, Wills EL, Halsey HJ (1975) Regional cerebral blood flow. Preliminary evaluation of an initial slope index in patients with unstable flow compartments. Stroke 6:142–148
10. Tytus JS, Seltzer HS, Kahn EA (1955) Cortisone as an aid in the surgical treatment of craniopharyngiomas. J Neurosurg 12:555–564
11. Weinstein JD, Toy FJ, Jaffe ME, Goldberg HI (1973) The effect of dexamethasone on brain edema in patients with metastatic brain tumors. Neurology 23:121–129

Use of Dexamethasone and Frusemide in Brain Edema Resulting from Brain Tumors

G. Meinig, H. J. Reulen, S. Wende, and K. Schürmann

Introduction

Referring to our previous papers [34, 35, 36, 40] concerning the treatment of peritumoral brain edema (BE) we have presented three possibilities for the assessment of antiedema treatment in brain tumor patients. By the use of these methods:

1. determination of water and electrolyte content in the peritumoral edema,
2. CT follow-up studies,
3. progress of neurological condition,

it is possible to estimate the quantitative effectiveness of different forms of antiedema treatment separately and in combination. This is important for the patient suffering from brain tumor since the antiedema treatment has to be adapted to the individual situation according to the presence or absence of symptoms of increased intracranial pressure (ICP), symptoms of impending herniation, as well as to the degree of peritumoral BE, the nature of the tumor, timing of craniotomy/biopsy (often determined by extrinsic factors) etc. In this study we have tested only two substances which are very important in antiedema therapy (apart from intensive care) namely, dexamethasone (D) and frusemide (F) as well as their combination (D/F). We will give a summary of our recent results and will try to draw some conclusions for the clinical situation – especially with respect to the three main aspects of the treatment of peritumoral edema:

a) preoperative treatment,
b) treatment during or after tumor extirpation,
c) long-term treatment of patients who cannot be operated on.

Materials and Methods

The following items were examined to assess the effect of antiedema treatment:

1. Change in water and electrolyte content: In the peritumoral area of 146 patients with a brain tumor. The following groups were compared:

I. 61 patients who did not receive any antiedema treatment served as control. This group contains 28 patients investigated by A. Baethman and P. Schmiedek (personal communication);
II. 29 patients who received dexamethasone in a dosage of 4×4 mg i.m./d for 4 to 6 days;

Treatment of Cerebral Edema
Edited by A. Hartmann and M. Brock

III. 11 patients who received 3×8 mg dexamethasone i.m. for 4 to 6 days;
IV. 11 patients who received 4×4 mg dexamethasone i.m. for a period of 2 to 4 weeks;
V. 34 patients treated with a combination of dexamethasone 4×4 mg i.m./d for 4 to 6 days and frusemide 3×40 mg post-op./d for 4 to 6 days;
VI. 18 patients given the combination treatment over a period of 2 to 4 weeks.

2. *Reduction of the area of peritumoral edema and of mass displacement* with the aid of CT in patients receiving the combined D/F therapy. The area of edema was estimated by planimetry, the reduction of midline shift was measured.

3. *Progress of neurologic condition* scored daily in 42 patients with a brain tumor treated with dexamethasone (4×4 mg i.m./d) using a special evaluation and documentation sheet (modified from [46] and [47]) (Table 1).

Table 1. Documentation sheet

Family name, first name
Date of birth
Age
Day of examination
Time of examination
State of consciousness
1. Normal
2. Responsive (slow in reaction)
3. Responsive (extremely slow in reaction)
4. Responsive to voice call, visual contact
5. Waking response to pain
6. Aimed defense reaction to pain
7. Unaimed defense reaction to pain
8. Flexion upon painful stimulation
9. Extensor spasm to painful stimulation
10. No response to painful stimulation

Orientation

A. Temporary orientation
   1. Normal
   2. Slightly impaired
   3. Severely impaired
   4. Lack of orientation

B. Local orientation
   1. Normal
   2. Slightly impaired
   3 Severely impaired
   4. Lack of orientation

Memory (recollection of recent events)
1. Normal
2. Slight
3. Severe
4. Total amnesia

Memory (recollection of distant events)
1. Normal
2. Slight
3. Severe
4. Total amnesia

Strength (contralateral to tumor)
1. Normal
2. Able to move against moderate resistance (slightly reduced function)
3. Able only to overcome gravity
4. Movement possible only when gravity counteracted
5. Pronounced paresis; contractions can only be seen or felt
6. Paralysis

Pupillary diameter (contralateral to tumor)
1. Extremely small
2. Small
3. Medium
4. Dilated
5. Maximally dilated

Pupillary reaction (homolateral to tumor)
1. Normal
2. Minimal
3. None

Babinski reflex (contralateral to tumor)
1. None
2. Suspicious
3. Positive

Babinski reflex (homolateral to tumor)
1. None
2. Suspicious
3. Positive

Results

1. Water and Electrolyte Content (Table 2; Figs. 1a, b)

Since we did not have the possibility of obtaining tissue samples of normal brain – as we were able to get from the peritumoral edematous brain tissue – we had to compare our findings of the water and electrolyte content of the edematous peritumoral area with the normal values given in the literature. However, the normal values of water content in cortex given by several authors [1, 15] are regularily said to be distinctly higher (at 84%) than our own values of peritumoral cortex (which might be edematous). This discrepancy is solved by Yates et al. [45], who pointed

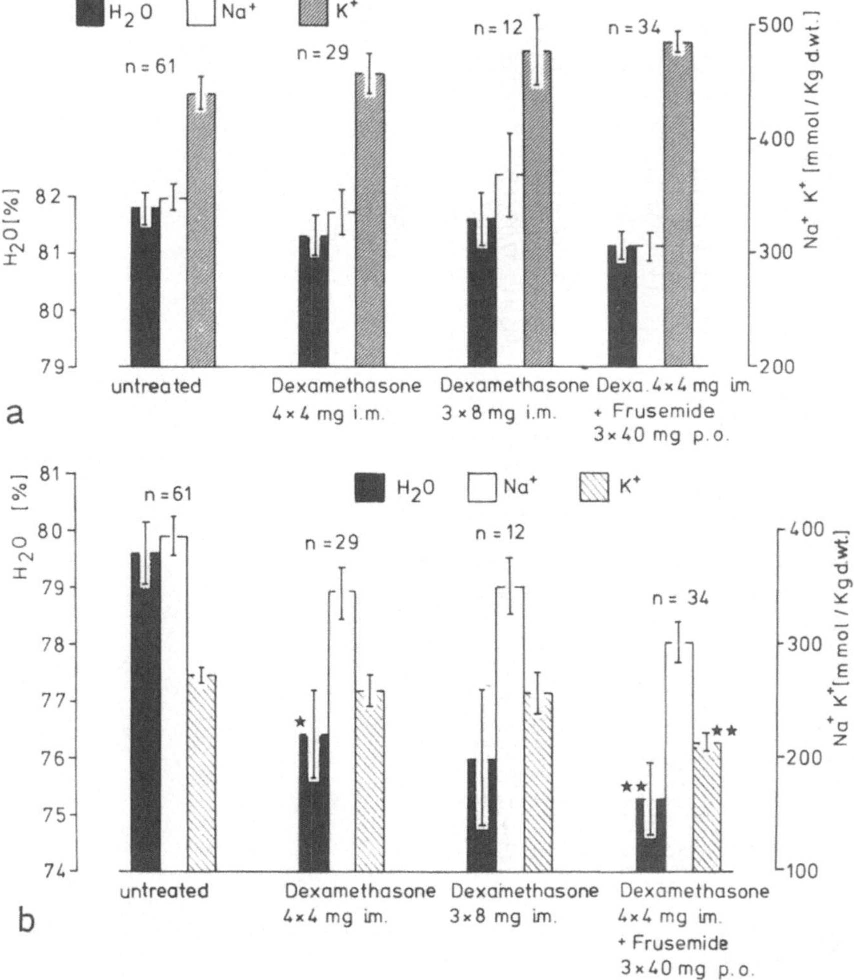

Fig. 1. a Water and electrolyte content in peritumoral area of cortex following different forms of antiedema therapy. **b** Water and electrolyte content in peritumoral area of edema of white matter following different forms of antiedema therapy

Table 2. Water and electrolyte content in peritumoral cerebral cortex and white matter in groups I to V

Measurement[a]	I	II	III	IV	V
Cerebral cortex					
H_2O	81.83 ± 0.30 (61)	81.31 ± 0.34 (29)	81.57 ± 0.47 (12)	81.98 ± 0.72 (11)	81.11 ± 0.26 (34)
Na	348 ± 12.60 (50)	334.90 ± 20.30 (27)	369.70 ± 38.60 (11)	357.20 ± 32.40 (11)	304.80 ± 13.70 (33)
Cl	301.10 ± 18.80 (13)	299.00 ± 27.20 (25)	345.80 ± 37.90 (11)	369.60 ± 34.60 (11)	324.00 ± 23.10 (33)
K	440.60 ± 13.70 (49)	457 ± 18.10 (27)	477.90 ± 30.80 (11)	496.80 ± 15.50 (11)	484.90 ± 8.40 (33)
White matter					
H_2O	79.61 ± 0.54 (61)	76.43 ± 0.80 (29)	75.95 ± 0.89 (12)	75.02 ± 1.46 (11)	75.24 ± 0.64 (34)
Na	389.33 ± 18.80 (47)	343.41 ± 23.37 (28)	350.12 ± 26.61 (12)	232.61 ± 36.46 (10)	306.92 ± 18.91 (33)
Cl	359.44 ± 27.32 (12)	304.85 ± 16.66 (26)	345.44 ± 37.08 (12)	335.65 ± 39.28 (10)	364.29 ± 26.55 (33)
K	272.32 ± 9.01 (48)	259.31 ± 13.97 (28)	260.68 ± 17.01 (12)	224.77 ± 9.50 (10)	212.47 ± 6.11 (33)

Note: Means ± SEM; number of patients in parentheses

[a] H_2O mg % milligrams percent, and electrolytes in milliequivalents per kilogram dry weight

out that there is a distinct increase of water content and change in the electrolyte concentration postmortem. Consequently these post-mortem high values are not comparable with our findings in the tissue biopsies taken from living patients. Sporadic examinations [45] of water content in cortex yield a value of 81.7% (normal cats 80.8%; dogs 80.1%). This is nearly the same value, which we found as an average in the peritumoral cortex of 61 patients (I.) who were not given any antiedema treatment. In any case it was not confirmed that BE really exists in peritumoral cortex. The assessment of pathological changes in water and electrolyte content of white matter is easier, since the postmortem changes are less marked than in the cortex. The values given in the literature for white matter range about 70.6% [1, 15]. Yates et al. [45] give a water content of normal white matter of 69.1% ($n=2$), if postmortem changes are eliminated (normal cats 68.2%; dogs 66.1%).

In any case the water content of white matter, which is comparable with our investigations, should lie about or below 70.0%. Since the average water content in peritumoral white matter of 61 patients was 79.61% (I.), an average increase of 10% results, if no antiedema treatment is given.

While the water content of the peritumoral cortex did not indicate significant BE and did not change significantly during antiedema treatment in the various groups (I.–VI.) – apart from a small diminution in the group which got D/F (group V) –, the tremendous pathological accumulation of water in the peritumoral white matter could be reduced more or less with respect to the various forms of therapy:

Group II. After treatment with D (4×4 mg i.m./d for 4–6 days) the water content decreased statistically significantly by nearly 2.5%.

Group III. After treatment with the higher dose of D (3×8 mg i.m./d for 4–6 days) the decrease of water content was nearly 3%.

Group V. after the combination therapy (D 4×4 mg i.m./d for 4–6 days and F 3×40 mg post-op./d for 2–6 days) the decrease of brain water content is nearly 4.5%.

Group IV. The same result can be obtained with a long-term treatment with D (4×4 mg i.m./d for 2–4 weeks).

Group VI. After long-term combination treatment we did not found a further reduction of BE.

However, as these patients suffered from huge tumors with massive shifts and severe accompanying illness, so that immediate trepanation had to be postponed, this group was not comparable with the others. The change in sodium content was in parallel with the changes in water content over a wide range. The potassium content did not change much after the therapy with D, but decreased in the cortex as well in one white matter after the combination therapy.

Stimulated by the clinical experience that the severity of brain edema as well as the results of treatment vary in accordance with the nature of the tumor, we have correlated the biochemical results with the nature of the brain tumor (Fig. 2). In the cortex the water content does not differ greatly between the treated and the untrated groups (only the small group of metastases shows a slightly increased water content). However, in the white matter the water content differs significantly in the different groups. It was highest in the untreated highly malignant tumors, glioblastomas and metastases. The results of treatment were not consistent in the group of semimalignant tumors and could not be prove in the group of the small number

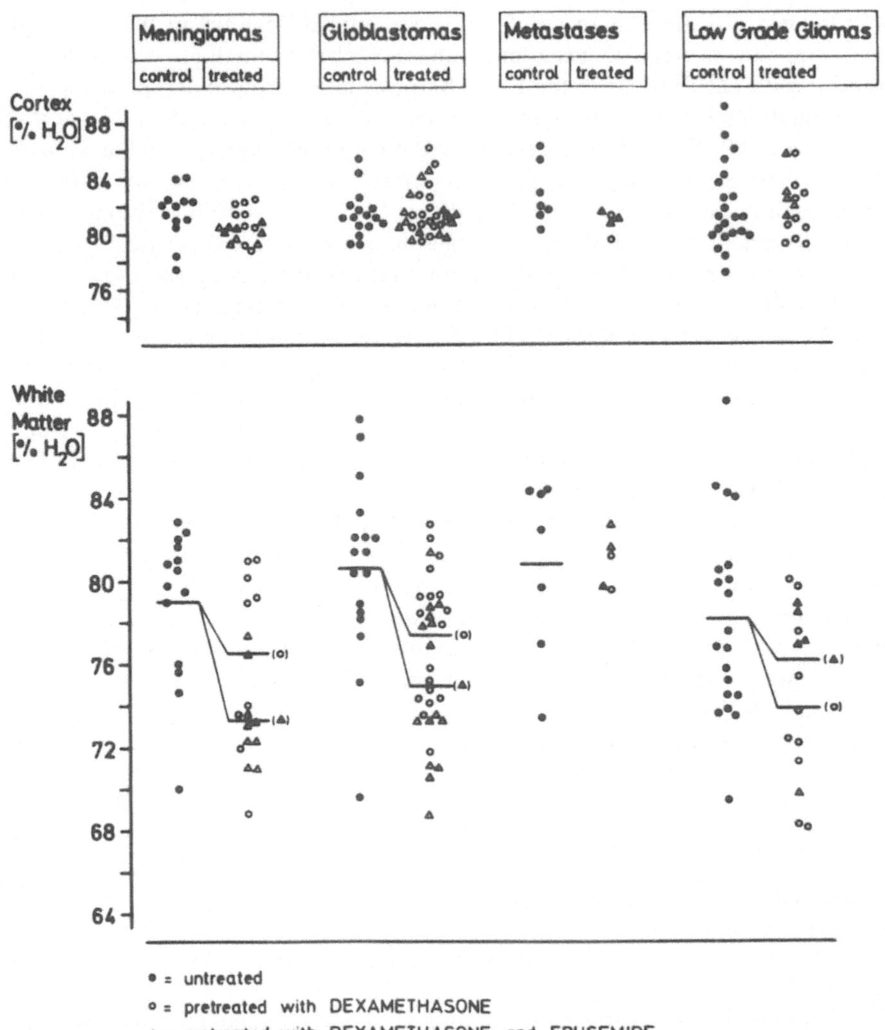

Fig. 2. Correlation of the result of antiedema therapy with the nature of respective brain tumors

of patients with metastases. The most marked reduction of edema compared to the untreated patient was found in the group of glioblastomas and meningiomas, where the decrease of water approaches 6% of water content.

2. Computerized Tomography (Follow-Up Study)

With some reservations, CT enables the dynamic process of formation and resolution of brain edema to be visualized. Figure 3 gives a typical example of extensive peritumoral brain edema in a case of suprasylvian glioblastoma. Three weeks after

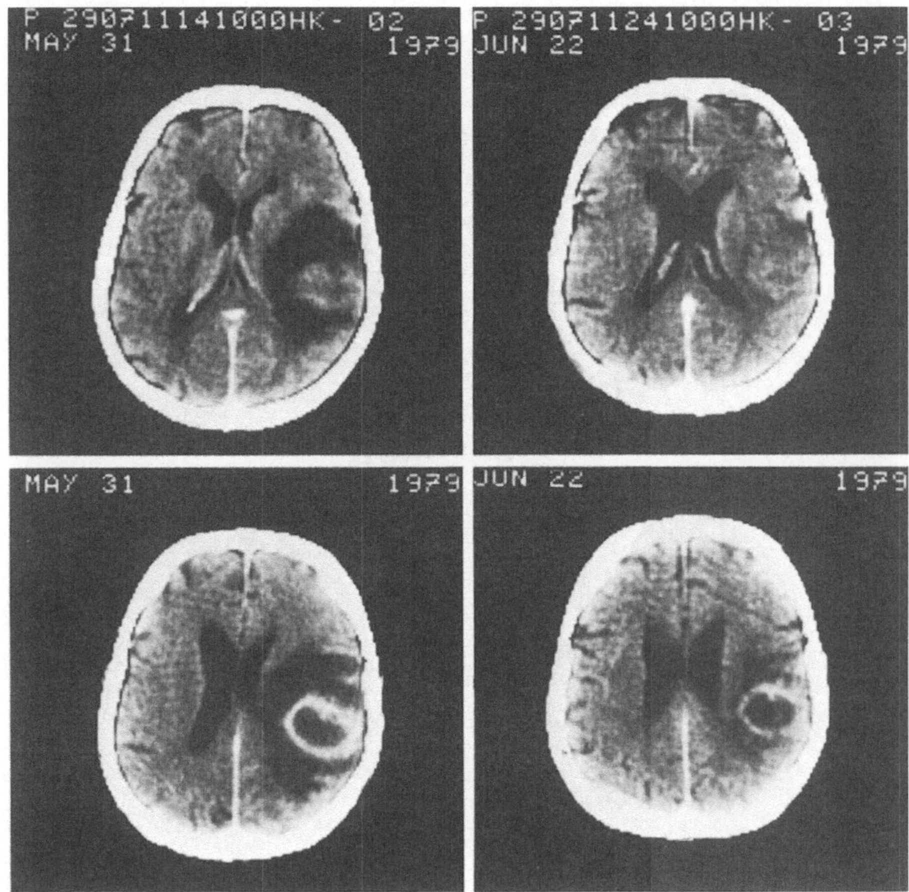

Fig. 3. CT showing decrease of peritumoral brain edema after therapy with 3×8 mg dexamethasone i.m./day over a period of 3 weeks

antiedema treatment with 3×8 mg dexamethasone i.m., the area of the brain edema has decreased significantly, the compressed lateral ventricle has reopened, and the midline shift has disappeared. We tried to measure the area of edema by planimetry. This is possible if the area of edema is well delineated and identical planes are available for comparison (of treated and untreated brain edema). Although estimating the boundary of the area of brain edema is partly subjective, various investigators reported basically the same results, with slight differences in the quantitative assessment. Figure 4a shows the diminution of the area of edema which was measured planimetrically during combination treatment with dexamethasone and frusemide in 20 patients. Nearly every patient showed a diminution of the area of edema during the combination treatment, although there were striking differences in the extent and the rate of the regression. These may depend on the nature of the tumor and its location. Further clarification of this question requires a large number of CT analyses. The reduction of the area of edema normally becomes apparent

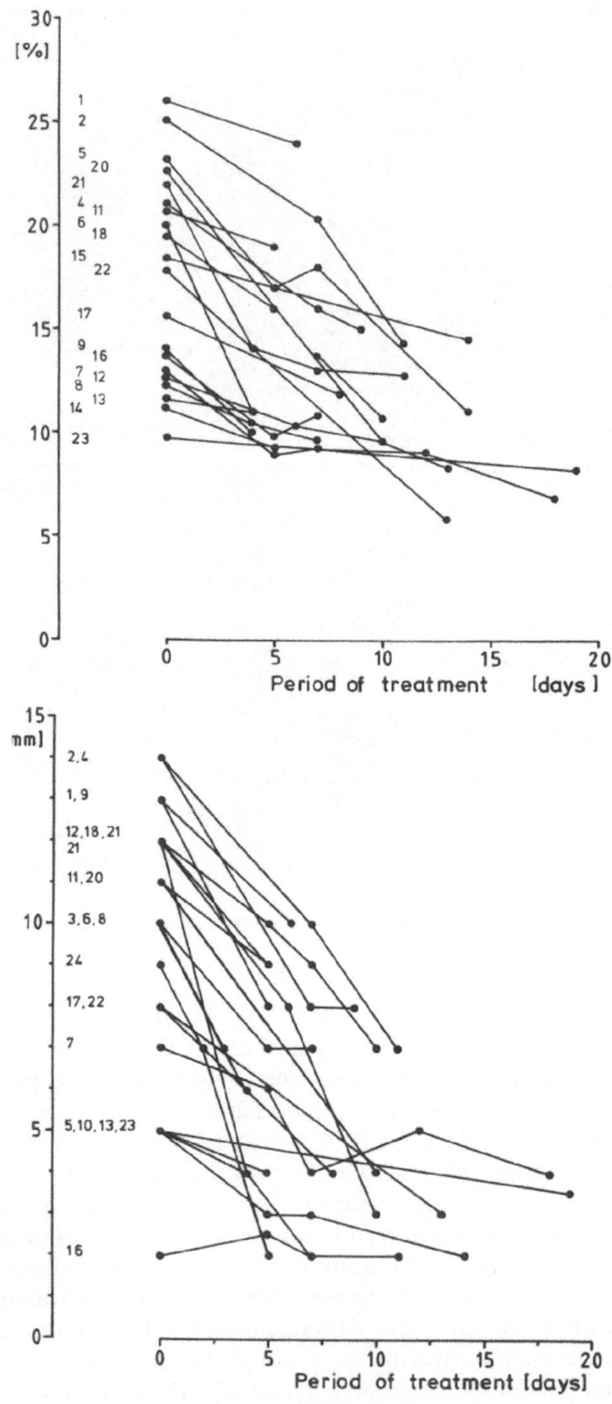

Fig. 4. a Diminution of edematous peritumoral area (evaluated planimetrically) during combination therapy with dexamethasone and frusemide. **b** Reduction of midline shift during combination therapy with dexamethasone and frusemide (Septum pellucidum)

within a few days, whereas neurological improvement sometimes requires only a few hours. The discrepancy may be explained by the limited resolution of the CT or by a direct effect of dexamethasone on the function of the brain cells, which may be independent of the antiedematous effect.

It is less difficult to determine the secondary changes due to brain edema, such as shifts of midline structures (septum pellucidum, pineal body, third ventricle, etc.), as well as the measurement of compressed cisterns, sulci and brain areas, and its regression. Figure 4 b shows the regression of the shift of the midline structure during the combination treatment in 22 patients (same groups as in Fig. 4 a). In principle, Fig. 4 b implies the same result as Fig. 4 a.

Table 3. Frequency distribution analysis before and after treatment with dexamethasone

				A. State of consciousness					
Grade of disorder	*1*	*2*	*3*	*4*	*5*	*6*	*7*	*(n)*[c]	*(nd)*[b]
Initial finding[c]	17	5	3	9	5	2	1	42	25
Final result[c]	37	5	–	–	–	–	–	42	5
				B. State of orientation					
Grade of disorder	*1*	*2*	*3*	*4*	*(n)*	*(nd)*			
Initial finding	19	1	8	14	42	23			
Final result	35	6	1	–	42	7			
				C. Memory (recollection of distant events)					
Grade of disorder	*1*	*2*	*3*	*4*	*(n)*	*(nd)*			
Initial finding	23	6	6	7	42	19			
Final result	38	4	–	–	42	4			
				D. Memory (recollection of recent events)					
Grade of disorder	*1*	*2*	*3*	*4*	*(n)*	*(nd)*			
Initial finding	19	2	10	11	42	23			
Final result	28	14	–	–	42	14			
				E. Paresis of the arm					
Grade of disorder	*1*	*2*	*3*	*4*	*5*	*6*	*(n)*	*(nd)*	
Initial finding	20	3	9	8	2	–	42	22	
Final result	31	8	1	1	1	–	42	11	
				F. Paresis of the leg					
Grade of disorder	*1*	*2*	*3*	*4*	*5*	*6*	*(n)*	*(nd)*	
Initial finding	20	4	9	7	2	–	42	22	
Final result	33	6	2	1	–	–	42	9	
				G. Babinski reflex					
Grade of disorder	*Neg.*	*Susp.*	*Pos.*	*(n)*	*(nd)*				
Initial finding	29	2	11	42	13				
Final result	35	5	2	42	7				

Note: *Neg.* negative; *Susp. suspicious; Pos. positive*

[a] *n* total patients

[b] *nd* neurological defects

[c] Initial finding before treatment. Final result after treatment

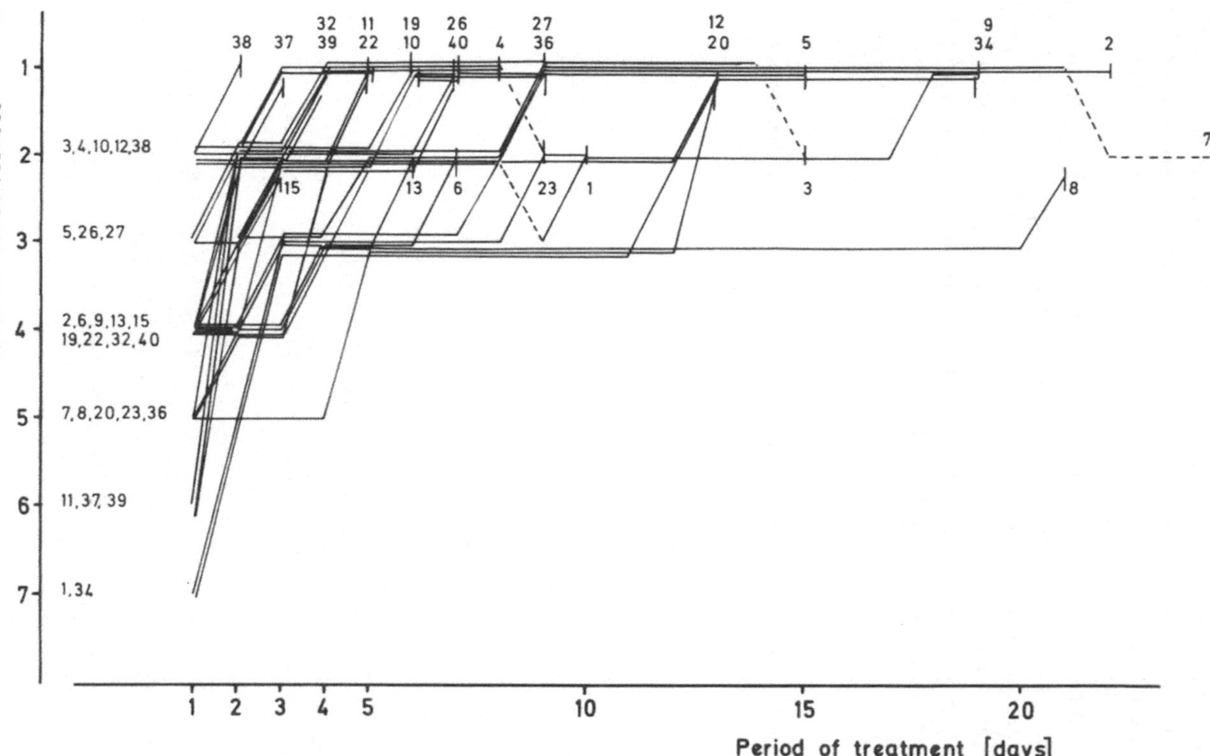

Fig. 5a. Improvement of state of consciousness during treatment with dexamethasone

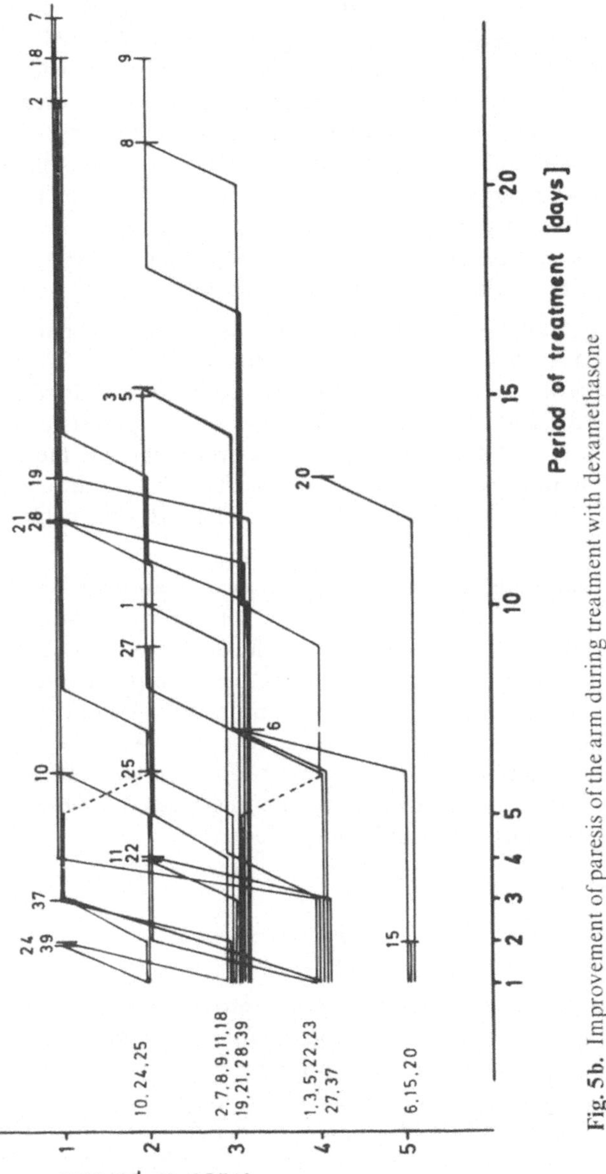

Fig. 5b. Improvement of paresis of the arm during treatment with dexamethasone

3. Progress of Neurological Condition

Analysis of the daily scoring of the neurological state during antiedema treatment with dexamethasone confirms the well-known fact that dexamethasone is able to reduce neurological disorders in brain tumor patients sometimes in a few hours [14, 26, 40]. A small group of patients with impending herniation who had to be operated on immediately was excluded from this study. No single symptom worsened upon dexamethasone treatment, and nearly all patients showed an improvement. However, the extent of the improvement of the neurological disorder differed considerably depending on the individual situation as well as with regard to the various different symptoms which were scored. Moreover, there were significant differences concerning the rate of the regression of the various neurological symptoms. The quantitative improvement of neurological disorders is illustrated by means of frequency distribution analysis before and after treatment with dexamethasone (Table 3). The frequency distribution for the various symptoms gives the extent of regression following the treatment period of six to nine days. Comparison of the symptoms investigated revealed significant differences in the final result.

Out of 25 patients (middle row, Table 3 A) with impaired consciousness 20 patients (lower row, Table 3 A) showed no disturbances after treatment and only five patients showed slight retardation of consciousness with slow reactions. On the other hand, among 22 patients (middle row, Table 3 E) with more or less paresis of the arm, only half (lower row, Table 3 E) showed complete recovery whereas the rest showed more or less incomplete improvement of the paresis. The disappearance of the Babinski reflex (Table 3 G) as well as the improvement of short-term memory (Table 3 D) showed a similar delayed tendency to improve.

Figure 5 a shows the extent of improvement for the disturbance of consciousness as well as its time dependence, and Fig. 5 b the same situation for improvement in the paresis of the arm. Although it is not possible to compare the degree of disturbance of these two symptoms, differences in the improvement of these symptoms are unmistakeable. The improvement of impaired consciousness improved after only a few hours of treatment whereas the paresis persisted in many cases for days. No single symptom worsened during the dexamethasone treatment if the initial finding is compared with the finding at the end of the dexamethasone treatment. We observed a secondary worsening after initial improvement in only a few cases.

Discussion

Our results confirm the well known fact, that D is able to improve neurological deficit in brain tumor patients, sometimes within a few hours. Until now a dose efficacy curve is still wanted. The time dependance of the improvement varies considerably depending on the individual situation, the various different symptoms which were scored, and the nature of the tumor and its location. Whether the D/F therapy is able to accelerate the improvement of neurological symptoms is still a question for further investigation. Our clinical impression is that the effect of D/F on neurological function is not much better than the treatment with D – except in the case of impending herniation. This is in line with the experimental studies of Pappius et al., 1972 [38] since D may accordingly influence cell metabolism and function directly in addition to its ability to help in the prevention and resolution of BE [40, 42]. Moreover the antiedema effect on peritumoral brain tissue as well of D [2, 14, 26, 33, 35, 40] as of F [38, 40, 41, 42[which is well known could be unequivocally confirmed. Our results show an additive effect of combination treatment with dexamethasone and frusemide. This may be explained by a different mode of action of the two drugs. It is postulated that among other mechanisms dexamethasone may decrease extravasation of edema fluid at the blood-brain barrier. On the other hand, diuretics such as frusemide and ethacrynic acid are known to reduce the rate of CSF production with a subsequent reduction of intracranial pressure. They may thus increase the clearance of edema fluid from the brain tissue to CSF [41, 42]. The reopening of the ventricles and probably of the subarachnoid space may be important factors in improving the clearance of edema fluid [41, 42].

It must be stressed, however, that the reduction of water content even in the peritumoral white matter is limited. Less than 50% of the pathological increase could be reduced maximally after longterm treatment for 2–4 weeks with D or D/F combination therapy of 2–6 days. Correspondently the CT follow-up studies showed only incomplete diminution of the area of decreased density (area of BE) and a preexisting significant midline shift never disappeared completely even after three weeks of D/ F therapy. If we compare the results of the neurological examinations and of the follow-up CT as well of the changes of water and electrolyte content in the peritumoral area – in order to establish the supposed relation BE/neurological deficit – we find beside good correspondence some controversial items: At first sight the reduction of neurological deficit runs parallel with the diminution of edema. On the other hand the chronological sequence does not coincide; we may have improvement of neurological disorder (especially in consciousness) within a few hours although BE may not be significantly diminished. We often observe complete neurological recovery but incomplete reduction of BE.

This leads to the question: Does BE directly cause neurological symtoms? R. D. Penn [39] and others doubt the direct influence. He refers to an experimental study by L. F. Marshall et al. [30], which showed that symptoms occur as the mass effect becomes important. As long as the ICP and CBF were normal the animals tolerated marked increases in brain water. Indeed the mass effect is a very important factor as R. A. Clasen et al. [6] also pointed out very impressively in stroke patients. They observed secondary brainstem hemorrhages when the weight increase of one hemisphere was 10–20% or more. Independent of the cause in a brain with a large mass lesion the pressure/volume curve may be in the steep part of its slope and a slight reduction in edema will be associated with marked improvement in neurological function. This is the one situation, where we observe the dramatic and rapid effect of D, which is related to the diminution of one secondary effect of BE, the reduction of increased ICP. It support the observations of Marshall and Penn [30, 39].

However, there are also hints which support the idea that there is a direct influence of BE on function. Frei et al. [11, 12] found a local rCBF decrease as well as local disturbance of energy metabolism in local BE induced by cold lesion without significant ICP increase. As a consequence focal neurological symptoms may occur. Moreover our own results concerning the improvement of neurological deficit does not have the only one aspect of quick rehabilitation of consciousness but also of delayed and incomplete improvement of several different symptoms which might be developed without any increase of ICP.

Until now we tend to believe that both situations exist: neurological deficit as a direct consequence of local BE and on the other hand of mass displacement and critically elevated ICP.

Therapeutic Consequences

a) Antiedema therapy given in the preoperative phase has the aim of improving the neurological deficit especially of reducing the complications caused by brain edema and increased ICP during and after the operation. The first point can be reached in many cases very easily, sometimes within a few hours at least as regards the improvement of impaired consciousness. The reduction of the water content in the peritumoral area, the reduction of ICP needs more strain and more time and until now is always incomplete. So the reduction of midline shift during treatment with dexamethasone is always incomplete even after two or three weeks and correlates with the reduction of the water content in the peritumoral area, which is maximally 50% after D/F-therapy for four to six days or a long-term treatment with D over a period of three weeks. This is only a limited result – which may be overlooked if the only good neurological improvement is considered. Severe BE during craniotomy – nowadays a rarity – or severe BE more frequently arising a few days postoperatively may often be caused by insufficient preliminary antiedema treatment.

Until now it is not easy to give a general valid plan of treatment, since every individual situation needs individual care, so that no global recommendation can be made. Since there was complete regression recovery from neurological deficits in a high percentage of patients within one week, treatment with dexamethasone (4×4 or 3×8 mg i.m./d) for several days or perhaps one week should be sufficient in most cases.

However, the CT follow-up studies and the results of the water and electrolyte evaluations, indicate that preoperative treatment should be much longer, especially if mass effects are obvious. The present study shows that it is possible to reduce significantly the length of preoperative treatment required, by treatment with dexamethasone and diuretics. Meanwhile we have administered in more than 150 patients 20 mg D/d perorally (4 mg tablet Decadron or Fortecortin) without any disadvantage.

The length of preoperative treatment is in any case limited by a secondary worsening of the neurological situation which sometimes occurs as early as a few days after starting antiedematous treatment (especially if the deficit is not caused by brain edema but by the brain tumor itself). Another criterion is that the antiedematous effect of dexamethasone and of diuretics may be exhausted after several weeks or months of administration. We have observed a few cases (unpublished) which received a long-term antiedematous treatment preoperatively for many weeks or several months. These patients reacted with massive brain edema during operation and (in particular) postoperatively. This massive edema could only be explained by the long-term treatment and the exhaustion of protective mechanisms against brain edema.

Since a maximal reduction of brain edema is desirable and the side effects of antiedema therapy are normally negligible and respond to therapy, we do not believe that there are serious objections to preoperative antiedema treatment lasting one to two weeks or in special situations several weeks.

b) Postoperative Treatment. BE during operation and postoperatively may be an activated peritumoral BE and is moreover a traumatic BE – which seems to be distinctly more refractory to therapy. Since moreover our investigations do not concern this form of BE, it is very difficult to give general recommendations for postoperative treatment. Our plan of treatment is geared to that of severe head trauma: To start with we give 24 to 100 mg dexamethasone i.v./d for a few days and reduce the dose step by step, if necessary we combine with frusemide e.g. 60 mg i.v. for a few days.

c) Long-Term Antiedema Therapy. Since the reduction of mass displacement and prevention of severe BE postoperatively is the most important point in patients, who are to be operated on, the long-term treatment in patients, who cannot be operated on has the aim of recovery from neurological deficit as complete as possible. On the other hand the dosage should be economical in order to have long lasting benefit of antiedema therapy.

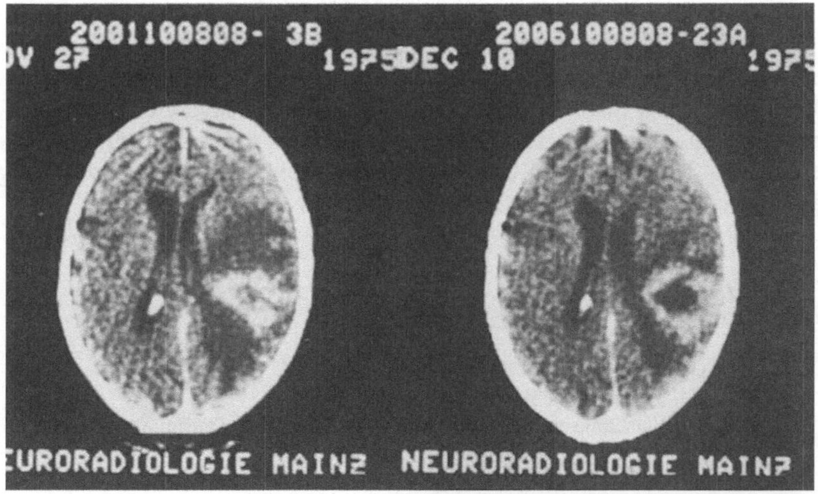

Fig. 6. Long-term CT study. Initially the patient received the combination therapy over a period of 2 weeks, and later he received 9 mg dexamethasone over a period of several months

The initial step of long-term treatment may be identical with the preoperative therapy. If the patient has improved and herniation does not threaten, the dose of D can be drastically reduced. In many cases 8 mg D/d is sufficient for many weeks or months. F can in most cases be stopped.
Figure 6 shows a typical example of long-term CT follow-up study. This patient initially received the combination therapy for two weeks, and later 9 mg dexamethasone per day p.o.
The patient was unconscious and showed a left-side hemiparesis when he was admitted to the clinic; he was fully conscious a few hours later, the hemiparesis disappeared during three days and six months later he showed no neurological deficit.
Initially we did not wish to administer the long-term combination therapy merely in order to complete our biochemical evaluation program. However, combination therapy was given in some cases because of clinical needs (severe brain edema, increase of intracranial pressure, severe accompanying illness) which delayed the immediate tumor extirpation. We were then able to determine the water and electrolyte content in a group of 18 patients (group VI. which was clinically not comparable with groups I.–V.). The therapeutic result of this retrospective determination was unfavorable. The water content was 76.83±0.84% [18], i.e. higher than in group V. This may be explained partly by the much more severe clinical situation. Moreover, the long-term antiedema effect may be exhausted after administration for several weeks. However, even this long-term combination therapy did not give rise to any side effects.

References

1. Adachi M, Feigin I (1966) Cerebral oedema and the water content of normal white matter. J Neurol Neurosurg Psychiat 29:446–450
2. Baethmann A, Lanksch W, Schmiedek P (1974) Formation and treatment of cerebral edema. Neurochirurgia 17, 37–47
3. Baethmann A, Oettinger W, Rothenfusser R (1977) Chemical mediator compounds in brain edema. Eur Surg Res 9:(Suppl. I), 121–122
4. Brock M, Wiegand H, Zillig C, Zywietz C, Mock P, Dietz H (1976) The effect of dexamethasone on intracranial pressure in patients with supratentorial tumors. In: Dynamics of brain edema. Pappius HM, Feindel W (eds). Springer, Berlin Heidelberg New York, pp 330–336
5. Clasen RA, Huchman MS, Pandolfi S, Laing I, Jacobs J (1976) Computed tomography of vasogenic cerebral edema. In: Dynamics of brain edema. Pappius HM, Feindel W (eds). Springer, Berlin Heidelberg New York, pp 278–282
6. Clasen RA, Huckmann MS, von Roenn KA, Pandolfi S, Laing I, Clasen JR (1980) Time course of cerebral swelling in stroke: A correlative autopsy and CT study. Advances in Neurology 28:395–412
7. Cserr HF, Cooper DN, Milhorat TH (1976) Production, circulation and absorption of brain interstitial fluid. In: Dynamics of brain edema. Pappius HM, Feindel W (eds)
8. Faupel G, Reulen HJ, Müller D, Schürmann K (1976) Double-blind study on the effects of steroids on severe closed head injury. In: Dynamics of brain edema. Pappius HM, Feindel W (eds). Springer, Berlin Heidelberg New York, pp 337–343
9. Faupel G, Reulen HJ, Müller D, Schürmann K (1978) Dexamethason bei schweren Schädel-Hirn-Traumen. Akt traumatol 8:265–281
10. Fenske A, Fischer M, Regli F, Hase U (1979) The response of focal ischemic cerebral edema to Dexamethasone. J Neurol 220:199–209

11. Frei HJ, Pöll W, Reulen HJ, Brock M, Schürmann K (1971) Regional energy metabolism, tissue lactate content and rCBF in cold injury edema. In: Brain and blood flow. Ross Russel RW (ed). Pitman Medical and Scientific Publishing Co, London, pp 125–129
12. Frei HJ, Wallenfang Th, Pöll W, Schubert R, Brock M (1973) Regional cerebral blood flow and regional metabolism in cold induced brain edema. Acta Neurochirurg 29:15–28
13. Gaab M, Knoblich OE, Schupp J, Dietrich K, Fuhrmeister U, Gruss P (1978) Wirkung unterschiedlicher Osmo- und Onkotherapie auf Hirndruck und elektrische Hirnaktivität beim experimentellen Hirnödem. Acta Neurochir 40:203–221
14. Galicich JH, French LA (1961) Use of dexamethasone in the treatment of cerebral edema resulting from brain tumors and brain surgery. Am Practitioner 12:169–174
15. Geigy wissenschaftliche Tabellen. 7. Auflage, p 515, 1968
16. Hadjidimos A, Brock M, Haas JP, Dietz H, Wolf R, Ellger M, Fischer F, Schürmann K (1969) Correlation between rCBF, angiography, EEG and Scanning in brain tumors. In: Cerebral blood flow. Springer, Berlin Heidelberg New York, pp 190–193
17. Hadjidimos A, Steingass U, Fischer F, Reulen HJ, Schürmann K (1973) The effect of dexamethasone on rCBF and cerebral vasomotor response in brain tumor. Eur Neurol 10:25–30
18. Hartmann A, Schütz HJ, Alberti E, Schreckenberger F, Loew F, Pycka J (1977) Effects of a new diuretic on Cerebrospinal Fluid Pressure in patients with supratentorial tumors. Arch Psychiat Nervenkr 224:351–360
19. Hartmann A, Alberti E (1977) Eine einfache Methode zur kontinuierlichen Messung des Liquordrucks. Acta Neurochir 36:201–214
20. Hartmann A, Alberti E (1977) Differentiation of communicating hydrocephalus and presenile dementia by continuous recording of cerebrospinal fluid pressure. J Neurol Neurosurg Psychiat 40:630–640
21. Hase U (1978) Intrakranielle Drucksteigerung. Neurochirurgia 21:145–157
22. Hase U, Reulen HJ, Meinig G, Schürmann K The influence of the decompressive operation on the intracranial pressure and the pressure-volume relation in patients with severe head injuries. Acta Neurochir (in press)
23. Klatzo I, Wisniewski H, Steinwall O, Streicher E (1967) Dynamics of cold injury edema. In: Brain edema. Klatzo I, Seitelberger F (eds). Springer, Wien New York, pp 554–563
24. Lanksch W, Oettinger W, Baethmann A, Kazner E (1976) CT findings in brain edema compared with direct chemical analysis of tissue samples. In: Dynamics of brain edema. Pappius HM, Feindel W (eds). Springer, Berlin Heidelberg New York, pp 283–287
25. Lanksch W, Kazner E (1976) CT findings in brain edema. In: Cranial Computerized Tomography. Lanksch W, Kazner E (eds). Springer, Berlin Heidelberg New York, pp 344–355
26. Long DM, Hartmann JF, French LA (1966) The response of human cerebral edema to glucosteroid administration. Neurology 16:521–528
27. Long DM, Maxwell RE, French LA (1971) The effects of glucosteroids upon cold induced brain edema. J Neuropathol Exp Neurol 30:680–697
28. Long DM, Maxwell RE, Choi KS, Cole HO, French LA (1972) Multiple therapeutic approaches in the treatment of brain edema induced by a standard cold lesion. In: Steroids and brain edema. Reulen HJ, Schürmann K (eds). Springer, Berlin Heidelberg New York, pp 87–94
29. Long DM, Maxwell RE, Choi KS (1976) A new therapy regimen for brain edema. In: Dynamics of brain edema. Pappius HM, Feindel W (eds). Springer, Berlin Heidelberg New York, pp 293–300
30. Marshall LF, Bruce DA, Graham DI (1976) Alterations in behavior, brain electrical activity, cerebral blood flow, and intracranial pressure produced by triethyl tin sulfate induced cerebral edema. Stroke 7:21–25
31. Marshall LF (1980) Treatment of brain swelling and brain edema in man. Advances in Neurology 28:459–469
32. Maxwell RE, Long DM, French LA (1971) The effects of glucosteroids upon cold-induced brain edema. In: Gross morphological vascular permeability changes. J Neurosurg 34:477–487
33. Maxwell RE, Long DM, French LA (1972) The clinical effects of a synthetic glucocorticoid used for brain edema in the practice of neurosurgery. In: Steroids and brain edema. Reulen HJ, Schürmann K (eds). Springer, Berlin Heidelberg New York, pp 219–232

34. Meinig G, Aulich A, Wende S, Reulen HJ (1976) Resolution of peritumoral brain edema following combination therapy with dexamethasone and furosemide. Adv Neurosurg 4:207–211
35. Meinig G, Aulich A, Wende S, Reulen HJ (1976) The effect of dexamethasone and diuretics on peritumor brain edema: Comparative study of tissue water content and CT. In: Dynamics of brain edema. Pappius HM, Feindel W (eds). Springer, Berlin Heidelberg New York, pp 301–305
36. Meinig G, Reulen HJ, Simon RS, Schürmann K (1980) Clinical, chemical and CT evaluation of short-term and long-term antiedema therapy with dexamethasone and diuretics. Advances in Neurology 28:471–489
37. Miller JD, Gudeman SK, Kishore PS, Becker DP (1980) Computed tomography in brain edema due to trauma. Advances in Neurology 28:413–422
38. Pappius HM (1972) Effects of steroids on cold injury edema. In: Steroids and brain edema. Reulen HJ, Schürmann K (eds). Springer, Berlin Heidelberg New York, pp 57–63
39. Penn RD (1980) Cerebral edema and neurological function: CT, evoked responses, and clinical examination. Advances in Neurology 28:383–394
40. Reulen HJ, Hadjidimos A, Schürmann K (1972) The effect of dexamethasone on water and electrolyte content and on rCBF in perifocal brain edema in man. In: Steroids and brain edema. Reulen HJ, Schürmann K (eds). Springer, Berlin Heidelberg New York, pp 239–252
41. Reulen HJ, Graham R, Fenske A, Tsuyumu M, Klatzo I (1976) The role of tissue pressure and bulk flow in the formation and resolution of cold-induced edema. In: Dynamics of brain edema. Pappius HM, Feindel W (eds). Springer, Berlin Heidelberg New York, pp 103–112
42. Reulen HJ, Graham R, Spatz M, Klatzo I (1977) Role of pressure gradients and bulk flow in dynamics of vasogenic brain edema. J Neurosurg 46:24–35
43. Schmiedek P, Guggemos L, Baethmann A, Lanksch W, Kazner E, Picha B, Oltenau-Nerbe V, Enzenbach R, Brendel W, Marguth F (1976) Re-evaluation of short-term steroid therapy for perifocal brain edema. In: Dynamics of brain edema. Pappius HM, Feindel W (eds). Springer, Berlin Heidelberg New York, pp 344–350
44. Thilmann J, Zeumer H (1974) Untersuchungen zur Behandlung des Hirnödems mit hohen Dosen Furosemid. Dtsch Med Wschr 99:932–935
45. Yates AJ, Thelmo W, Pappius HM (1975) Post-mortem changes in the chemistry and histology of normal and edematous brains. Am J Pathol 79:555–564
46. Begleitblatt und Verlaufskontrolle für Schädel-Hirnverletzte (6. Aufl.) (Faupel et al.)
47. Verlaufskontrollblatt für die Neurochirurgische Intensivstation, deployed by Arbeitsgruppe “Schädel-Hirntrauma” der Deutschen Gesellschaft für Neurochirurgie

Effect of Dexamethasone on Regional Cerebral Blood Flow in Ischemic Cerebral Infarction

A. Hartmann, J. Menzel, and C. Buttinger

In the acute state of ischemic apoplexy brain edema leading to increase of intracranial pressure and reduction of regional cerebral blood flow (rCBF) plays an important role [17, 19]. At present hyperosmolar solutions are recommended for treatment of brain edema of ischemic nature whereas the value of steroids is debated [13, 21]. Clinical results are conflicting. Experimental studies (Table 1) have used different models, species, mode of production of infarction, doses of steroids and parameters [2, 3, 4, 5, 7, 8, 10, 12, 15, 25]. Only two studies evaluate the effect of dexamethasone on rCBF in the presence of cerebral ischemia [2, 3]. Both studies do not measure rCBF for longer than 24 hours.

Since the effect of chronic administration of dexamethasone on rCBF in animals suffering from regional cerebral ischemia is not known but might be important for further evaluation we have conducted the following study:

Method

Nineteen baboons of both sexes with a mean weight of 12 kg completed the protocol. After initial intravenous anesthesia with pentobarbital sodium (20 mg/kg) and intubation anesthesia was performed with a gas mixture of 75% nitrous oxide and 25% oxygen. Muscular relaxation was achieved with repeated injections of suxamethonium. The first rCBF-studies proved normal autoregulation and blood gas reactivity.

Body temperature was controlled by using a heat matress. Continuous recording of systemic blood pressure and central venous pressure was performed after catheterization of the femoral artery and vein. Blood gases were checked regularily by a gas analyser, using the arterial blood.

For measurement of rCBF on the first day a polyethylene catheter with an outer diameter of 1 mm was introduced into the lingual artery, the tip at the origin of this vessel. All other vascular branches of the common carotid artery except the internal carotid artery were temporarily ligated.

On the other days of rCBF-measurements other branches of the common carotid artery were used for introduction of the catheter with ligation of the rest of the branches. By this procedure it was ensured that Xenon 133 entered only the internal carotid artery. At the end of each rCBF-day the catheter was removed, the artery used permanently ligated and all other vessels opened again.

For measurement of rCBF and neurosurgical intervention the baboon was placed in a stereotactic frame. Since the collimator, holding the detectors, was fixed to the

Treatment of Cerebral Edema
Edited by A. Hartmann and M. Brock

Table 1. Studies which evaluated effect of dexamethasone on experimental cerebral ischemia

Author	Year	Animal	Values measured	Dose	Length of study	Production of cerebral ischemia	Interpretation of effect
Plum et al.	1963	Rat	Mortality	0.55 mg/kg 1.1 mg/kg	1 day	Carotid ligation and anoxic exposure	Negative
Harrison and Russel	1972	Gerbil	Mortality	5 mg/kg/day	2 days	Common carotid artery (CCCA) ligation	Positive
Kahn et al.	1972	Gerbil	Clinical course, Mortality	0.5 mg/kg/day	Not indicated	CCA ligation	Positive
Bartko et al.	1972	Cat	rCBF, Metabolism Edema fluid	0.3 mg/kg/day before infarction	2 hours	Middle cerebral artery (MCA) occlusion	Positive
Siegel	1972	Rat	Electrolytes mortality	1 mg/kg/day	3 days	Microemboli	Negative
Harrison et al.	1973	Gerbil	Mortality, Water content	5 mg/kg/day	2 days	CCA ligation	Positive
Donley and Sundt	1973	Squirrel monkey	Clinical course, Pathology	0.14 mg/kg 0.075 mg/kg	2 days	MCA ligation	Negative
Lee et al.	1974	Cat	Clincal course, Pathology	4 mg/kg/day	2 weeks	MCA ligation	Negative
Hoppe et al.	1974	Cat	Clinical course, Water content	4 mg/kg	2 days	MCA ligation	Positive
De la Torre and Surgeon	1976	Rhesus monkey	Clinical course, dry/wet Weight rCBF	unclear: 12 mg/kg for 1 day (?)	7 days	MCA ligation for 17 hours	Negative
Fenske et al.	1979	Cat	Edema fluid, Electrolytes, Blood-brain-barrier, Mortality	2.55 mg/kg	1 day	MCA ligation	Positive

frame, rCBF-desaturation curves were always recorded from identical regions of interest.

After the first rCBF-run ischemic infarction was produced by clipping the left middle cerebral artery using the transorbital approach [18, 26]. After the clip was placed the orbital cavity was filled with dental cement (Fig. 1). Thus the animal could be kept in the cage for weeks.

rCBF was measured by the intra-arterial Xenon 133 method. Eight NaJ-detectors were placed in a lead collimator fixed to the stereotactic frame. The diameter of the crystal was 8 mm, collimation was 10–14 mm. Xenon 133 in a dose of 0.8–1.5 mCi was injected into the lingual catheter. Clearance curves were recorded for 17 minutes, stored on paper tape and processed in a Hewlett Packard computer. The stochastic method was used. Correction of the Xenon 133 partition coefficient was done according to hemoglobin measurements. Since the study was performed controlled (treated and non-treated group) it was assumed that any alteration of the partition coefficient was the same in both groups. Basal rCBF was the steady state rCBF in each animal and each region prior to positioning of the clip calculated for $PaCO_2$ of 40 mm Hg using the individual regional blood gas reactivity factor (RF). RF was calculated from normocapnic and hypercapnic rCBF-measurement, using changes of rCBF and $PaCO_2$.

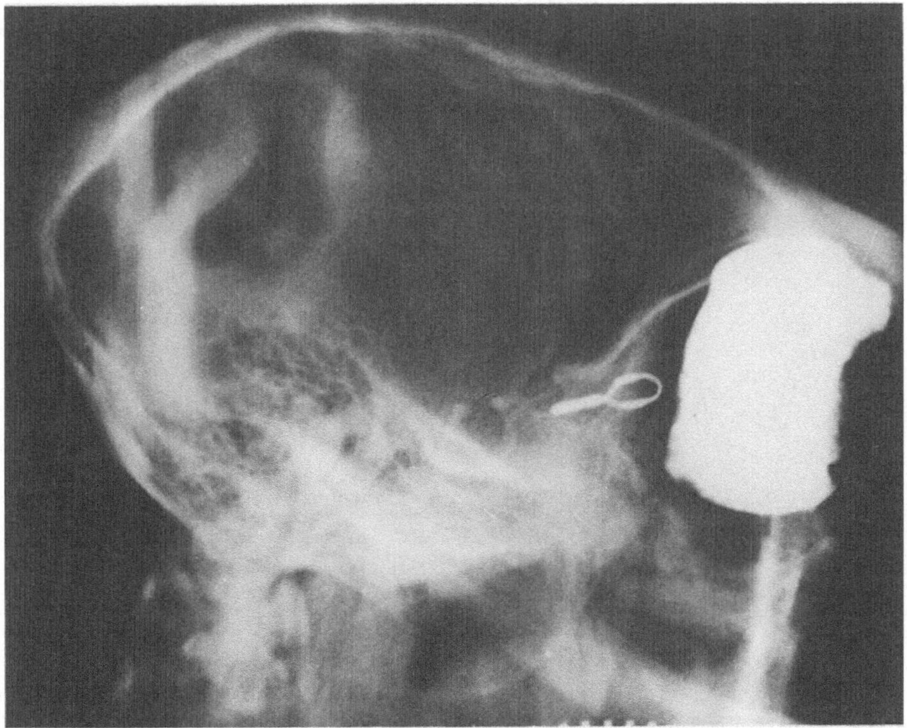

Fig. 1. Skull X-ray of a baboon. Middle cerebral artery clip and dental cement in the orbital cavity are shown

Each rCBF-run consisted of:

a) steady state measurement during normal blood pressure and normocapnia ($PaCO_2$ between 32 and 38 mm Hg)
b) hypercapnia ($PaCO_2$ between 48 and 54 mm Hg) and normal blood pressure
c) hypotension with systemic blood pressure between 80 and 95 mm Hg and normocapnia (autoregulation test).

After the first rCBF-run the clip was positioned. One hour and four hours later rCBF-run 2 and 3 were performed. rCBF-run 4 was done on the 7th day and rCBF-run 4 on the 28th days after the infarction was produced.
Six animals were treated with dexamethasone in the following doses: 1 mg/kg/day for 10 days, thereafter with reduced doses till the 13th day. From day 14 till day 28 these animals were not treated. Treatment was started one hour after positioning of the clip. The control group (13 animals) was not treated with dexamethasone. The selection of animals was randomized.

Results

None of the animals in the treated group died during the protocol of 28 days.
Two of the control animals died before the 7th day, five after the 7th day and six control animals survived.
None of the (treated and non-treated) baboons had loss of consciousness for longer than 24 hours. All animals developed a right-sided faciobrachial hemiparesis of varying degree with no recognizable difference of intensity between the two groups. None of the animals which survived was free of neurological symptoms on the 28th day of the study. Between both groups there was no significant difference for blood gases, blood pressure, hemoglobin and pH.

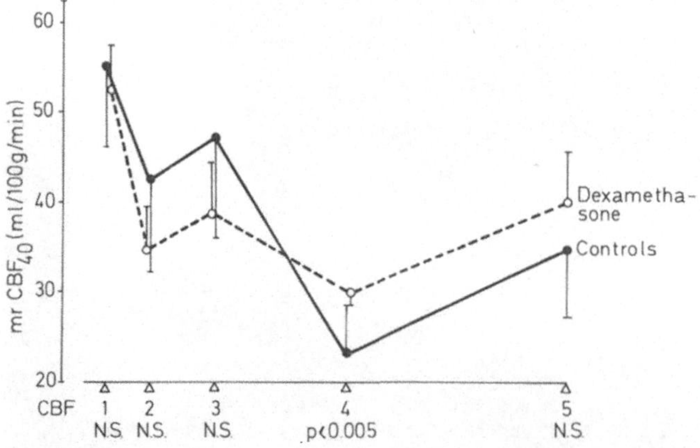

Fig. 2. Mean regional cerebral blood flow (mrCBF) in ml/100 g/min during course of the study. All treated and nontreated animals which were alive at the time of each CBF-run 1–5 were included in calculation of the flow data. *N.S.* no significant difference between dexamethasone and control group; *p* level of significance

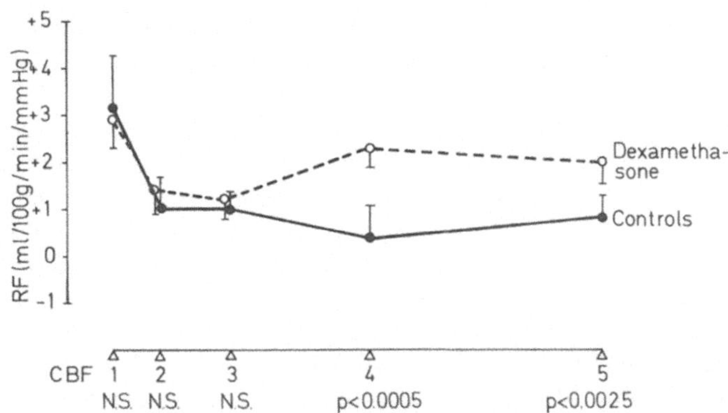

Fig. 3. Mean regional blood gas reactivity factor RF in ml/100 g/min/mm Hg during course of the study. RF indicates change of rCBF per mm Hg of altered $PaCO_2$ during hypercapnia. Abbreviations as in Fig. 2

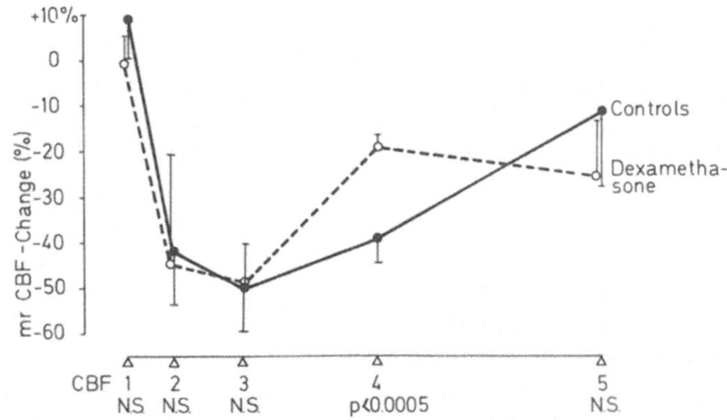

Fig. 4. Mean regional autoregulation in % during course of the study. Autoregulation is expressed as %-change of mean rCBF during systemic hypotension compared to steady state rCBF during normotension. Abbreviations as in Fig. 2

Figures 2–4 indicate blood flow, blood gas reactivity factor RF and autoregulation of both groups. The data contain values of those animals which were alive at the time of the measurement independent whether they died later during the protocol or not. F.i. data of rCBF run 4 (day 7) include the measurements of control animals which died by the 28th day.

Figure 2 indicates that mean regional cerebral blood flow (mean rCBF) dropped in both groups immediately after positioning of the clip, increased slightly four hours later and decreased further seven days after clip positioning (c.p.), but 28 days after c.p. there was slight improvement of mean rCBF. However, normal values were not reached. Luxury perfusion with mean rCBF above steady state value (CBF 1) was never observed [31]. In none of the cases mean rCBF fell below 17 ml/100 g/min.

Only seven days after c.p. there was a significant difference between both groups: the treated group showed a higher mean rCBF than the control group ($p < 0.005$).

Figure 3 indicates that mean regional blood gas reactivity factor RF decreased in both groups to the same degree immediately after c.p. There was no change four hours later (CBF-run 3). Seven and 28 days after c.p. RF decreased to the same extent in the control group but was significantly higher in the dexamethasone-group. RF in the group on day 7 and day 28 was almost normal compared to CBF-run 1. Blood flow autoregulation (Fig. 4) is expressed as percentage reduction of mean rCBF during blood pressure hypotension (above physiological limit of autoregulation, which is about 80 mm Hg) compared to the mean rCBF value during normotension (steady state). All animals had normal autoregulation during CBF-run 1. After c.p. autoregulatory capacity decreased to 45–50% in both groups and remained unchanged during CBF-run 3 (4 hours after c.p.). Thereafter it increased in both groups till day 7 but significantly faster in the dexamethasone-group. On day 28 autoregulatory capacity was disturbed in both groups but less in the control animals.

Regional Data

Eight detectors recorded clearance curves from the left hemisphere. Steady state rCBF during CBF-run 1, regional RF and autoregulation index were normal and identical for both groups, independent whether some of the control animals died later on during their course or not. rCBF during steady state was highest in the frontal lobe and lowest in the occipital lobe. RF was high over the frontal, parietal and occipital lobe and lower over the temporal and precentral aspect [28]. There were no differences between the regional autoregulatory capacities [27, 29].
The eight detectors were grouped according to the location and the distribution of the three main cerebral arteries. The three perfusion territories represented flow in the area of the anterior (ACA), middle (MCA), and posterior (PCA) cerebral artery. Figure 5 indicates rCBF-alteration in both groups. In the MCA-territory rCBF dropped immediately after c.p. and did not recover. There was no significant differ-

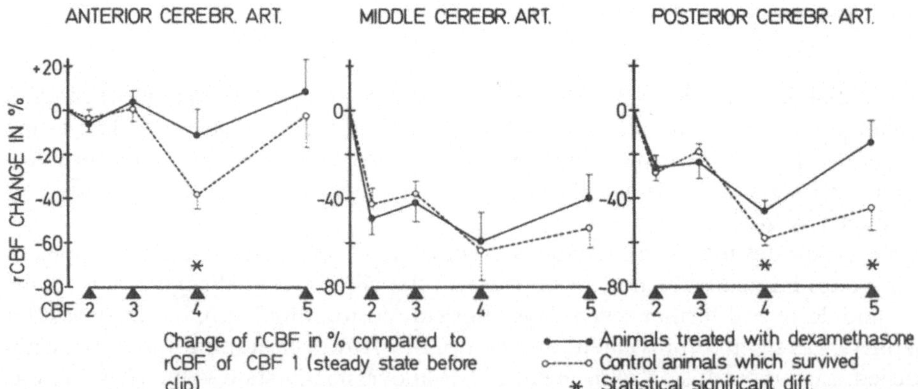

Fig. 5. Change of rCBF in different perfused areas during course of the study. rCBF expressed as %-difference between flow data of CBF-run 2 – 5 to that of CBF-run 1. For the Figs. 5–7 only treated and untreated animals which survived the protocol (CBF-run 1–5) were included

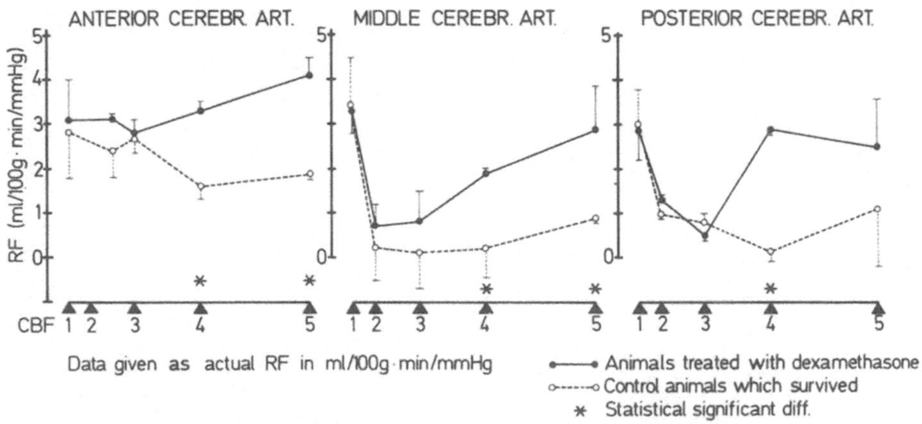

Fig. 6. Change of blood gas reactivity factor RF during course of the study

ence between the two groups. There was no difference from the first to the fourth hour after c.p. but an additional reduction from day one till day seven. In some animals (both, controls and treated ones) rCBF on day seven fell below 15 ml/100 g/min. On day 28 rCBF in the dexamethasone group was slightly better than in the untreated animals. However, the difference did not reach level of significance.

rCBF in the territory of the ACA was normal for the total protocol in the dexamethasone group. In the control group rCBF in this area was normal on day one but reduced for almost 40% on day seven. Twenty-eight days after c.p. rCBF was normal again. In the territory of the PCA rCBF decreased one hour after c.p., remained unchanged reduced during CBF-run 3 and decreased further till day 7. However, in the treated baboons flow reduction was less. On day 28 rCBF decrease in the control animals was greater than the dexamethasone animals.

Blood gas reactivity (Fig. 6) in the territory of the MCA was reduced from CBF-run 2–5 in the control group. In some animals RF reached negative values on the day of infarction and on day 7. This indicates complete vasoparalysis with intracerebral steal phenomenon (blood flow reduction during hypercapnia). Complete vasoparalysis was never observed in the dexamethasone group, not even during the early phase of infarction. From day one till day seven there was an improvement of RF in the treated group with a significant difference to the control group. On day 28 RF in the animals treated with steroids was almost normal. Again there was a significant difference from the control animals.

In the territory of the ACA regional RF was always normal in the dexamethasone group. In the control group RF was not changed during the early phase of infarction (run 2 and 3) but reduced on day 7, and 28 days post c.p. RF was identical to day 7.

In the territory of the PCA RF was grossly impaired in both groups immediately after c.p. and four hours after c.p. there was no change. On the day 7 and 28 RF was decreased in the control animals, again with complete vasoparalysis in some animals. In the treated animals RF became normal from day one till seven and remained normal on day 28. A significant difference between both animals groups was observed only on day seven.

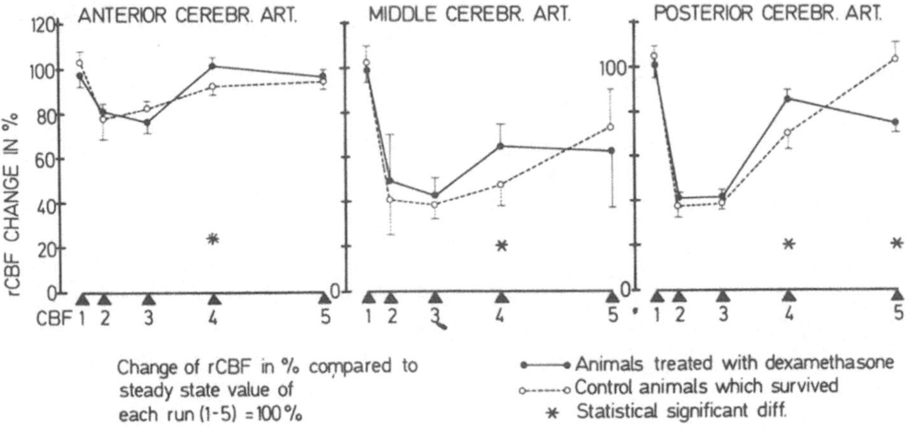

Fig. 7. Change of autoregulatory capacity during course of the study

Autoregulation (Fig. 7) was impaired in the territory of the MCA in both groups for the total time of the study. It decreased a short time after the start of ischemia and thereafter increased slightly till day seven. However, on day seven autoregulation was better in the treated group, but 28 days after c.p. there was no difference between both groups.

The territory of the ACA showed slightly impaired autoregulation for both groups on day one and improvement thereafter. The treated animals showed a better recovery with normal autoregulation. On day 28 autoregulation was normal in both groups.

The territory of the PCA presented with the same degree of damage to autoregulatory mechanism for both groups on day one. The degree of impairement was the same as in the territory of the MCA. Till day seven autoregulation improved in the

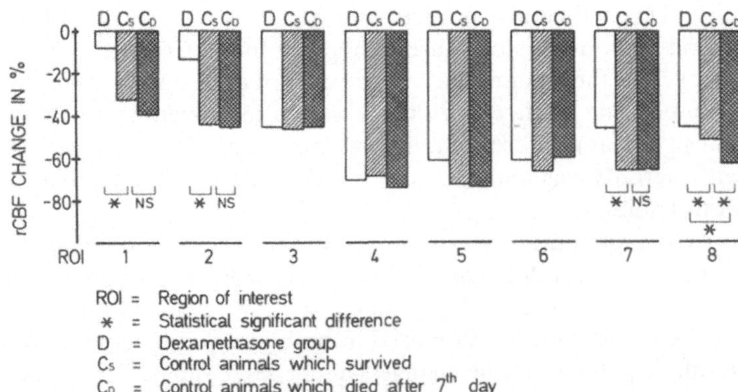

Fig. 8. Change of rCBF in all 8 areas between rCBF before c.p. and 7 days after c.p. rCBF-change indicated as %-alteration from CBF-run 1 to CBF-run 4. A significant difference between control animals which survived (C_S) and control animals which died between 7th and 18th day (C_D) was observed in ROI 8 (PCA)

PCA-area in both groups but more in the dexamethasone group and 28 days after c.p. autoregulation was better in the untreated than in the treated animals.

Considering all observations it became obvious that the most prominent alterations of all parameters and the biggest differences between treated and untreated animals occurred on day 7 (CBF-run 4). This involved all territories. The following figures compare the data of each single region of interest between steady state (CBF-run 1) and day 7 (CBF-run 4) and include values of those animals which died after the seventh day.

Figure 8 compares rCBF-data of each region and indicates that there was a significant difference regarding flow data of region of interest (ROI) 1, 2 (both ACA) and 7, 8 (PCA) between control and treated animals. This higher reduction of rCBF concerns both, control animals which survived and control animals which died after day seven. In addition to that rCBF in ROI 8 (PCA) of the baboons which died was lower than that of the surviving animals.

Figure 9 indicates RF differences between CBF-run 1 and CBF-run 4 for all three groups. Except ROI 5 (MCA) all areas in the control animals had a lower reactivity to alteration of blood gases than those of the dexamethasone animals. In ROI 5 reactivity of the animals which died was significantly lower than that of the surviving control and dexamethasone animals. In addition RF of the dying baboons was significant lower than RF of the surviving control animals for area 1 (ACA), and 7 (PCA).

Similar observations were done for the autoregulation (Fig. 10). In the territory of the MCA (ROI 3–6) change of autoregulatory capacity was worse for the control animals than for the treated animals in all but one ROI with no difference between dying and surviving animals. In the territory of the ACA and PCA recovery from

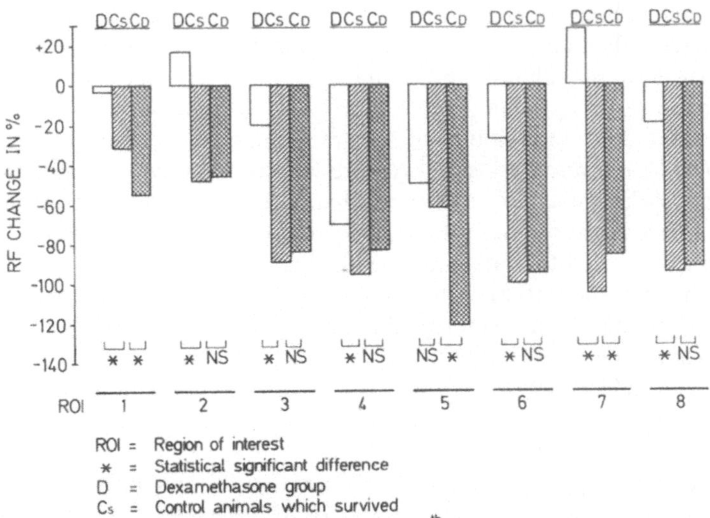

Fig. 9. Change of blood gas reactivity factor RF in all areas from CBF-run 1 to CBF-run 4. Change of RF is expressed as %-alteration from RF of CBF-run 1 to RF of CBF-run 7. A significant difference between C_S and C_D was observed in ROI 1 (ACA), 5 (MCA) and 7 (PCA)

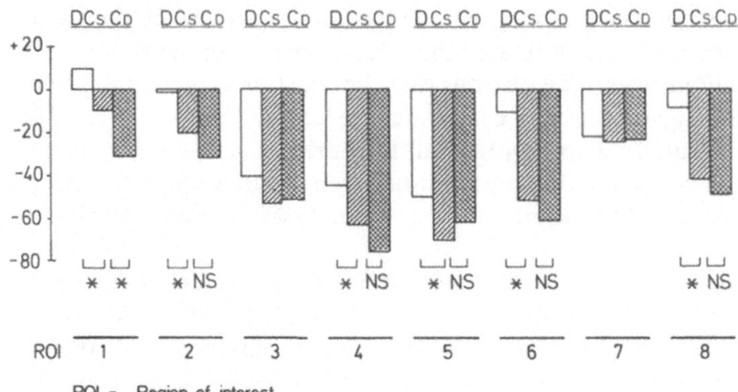

Fig. 10. Change of autoregulatory capacity between CBF-run 1 and CBF-run 4 for all 8 areas, expressed as %-alteration from CBF-run 1 (=100%). A significant difference between surviving (C_S) and dying (C_D) control animals was observed in ROI 1 (ACA)

damage to autoregulation was worse for the control animals compared to the treated animals. Further, improvement of autoregulation in ROI 1 (ACA) was worse for the animals which died than that for the surviving animals.

Discussion

Studies about courses of ischemic developed edema indicate that fluid accumulation starts early after production of ischemia [5, 11, 14, 16, 20]. Reduction of blood flow, loss of autoregulation and damage to blood gas reactivity occur a short time after the start of infarction [1, 7, 9, 20, 22, 23, 29] and can be observed over a prolonged period [30]. Acute failure of substrate delivery, metabolism, reactivity to change of blood gases and perfusion pressure with consecutive accumulation of intra- and extracellular water are important factors for the clinical deficit. Inhibition of further damage is important for the course and outcome of the victim.

We have tried to imitate a clinical situation and started with steroid therapy a short time after the start of ischemia and administered it over a prolonged period.

The model which was selected guaranteed a reproducible localised ischemia leading to neurological deficit with a typical faciobrachial paralysis. The baboon has a cerebral vascular architecture which is similar to that of the human. In contrast to the cat the tentorium is not bony in nature so that changes of the intracranial pressure are comparable to those in the human.

The use of a stereotactic frame for fixation of both animals and collimator provides a reproducible "view" of the detector to the tissue cylinder of interest. The intra-arterial Xenon 133-technique bears problems like recirculation, non- homogenous initial filling of the tissue, crosstalk via crossfilling, unknown partition coefficient and diffusion from high- to low-concentrated areas. Still it is the most reliable method for measuring regional cerebral blood flow of larger tissue areas over a prolonged time.

Regarding the spontaneous course of rCBF it became obvious that initial reduction of flow is confined to the area of the MCA directly involved (Fig. 5). Till the seventh day rCBF reduction involves the neighboring areas of the unclipped ACA and PCA thus indicating spread of edema [6]. Blood gas reactivity and autoregulation were impaired in perifocal areas from the very first moment (Figs. 6, 7). With reduction of flow in the ACA/PCA-territory at the end of the first week (day 7, CBF-run 4) blood gas reactivity worsened but autoregulation improved. This slight improvement in the perifocal areas was observed also in the directly involved area of the MCA.

The prolonged damage to blood gas reactivity in perifocal tissue areas despite partial normalization of flow (ACA) and complete normalization of autoregulation (ACA and PCA) might be explained by the maturation phenomenon [14] which leads to progressive damage in the presence of restored perfusion. This again might be influenced by the development and spread of edema to areas which do not suffer from primary ischemia. Dexamethasone has proved in this study that it supports recovery from acute reduction of cerebral blood flow (Fig. 2) and prevents further decrease of flow from the acute to the chronic state (Fig. 2, CBF-run 4). At the same time it prevents (ACA) and impairs (PCA) reduction of flow in the perifocal tissue during the subchronic phase.

Dexamethasone did not affect blood flow in the ischemic area itself (Fig. 5, MCA). Still it had some beneficial action on this territory and on its blood flow regulation since blood gas reactivity and autoregulation were improved (Figs. 6, 7). Parallel to prevention of rCBF-drop of the perifocal ACA-area the administration of this steroid did improve blood gas reactivity and autoregulation.

In this experiment dexamethasone did not affect the values on the day of infarction (till four hours after clip positioning). This might be explained by the hypothesis that the cytotoxic state of ischemic edema is not influenced but its transition to vasogenic state.

We do not have any explanation why autoregulation in the PCA-territory was normal at the end of the protocol in the control group but not in the treated group. However, this was the only drawback, observed during the protocol. It cannot be excluded that the period of dexamethasone therapy was too short.

One of the most striking differences between both groups was the fact that none of the animals treated with dexamethasone died, but seven out of 13 control baboons did. The study was designed according to a randomized selection and performed until six animals in each group survived the four-week period of observation. Separating the data of the surviving (C_S) from those of the dying (C_D) control animals it was indicated that blood flow in C_D-group fell more till the 7th day in the PCA-area but not in the MCA-territory. Blood gas reactivity in the C_D-group was worse compared in the C_S-animals in some of both, focal and perifocal areas. Autoregulation was worse only in one region of the animals which died after the seventh day. Since these differences between dying and surviving control baboons were not observed on the day of infarction (including those which died between day one and day seven), it might be speculated that dexamethasone might prevent fatal outcome after infarction by protecting CBF-regulation. In summary we conclude

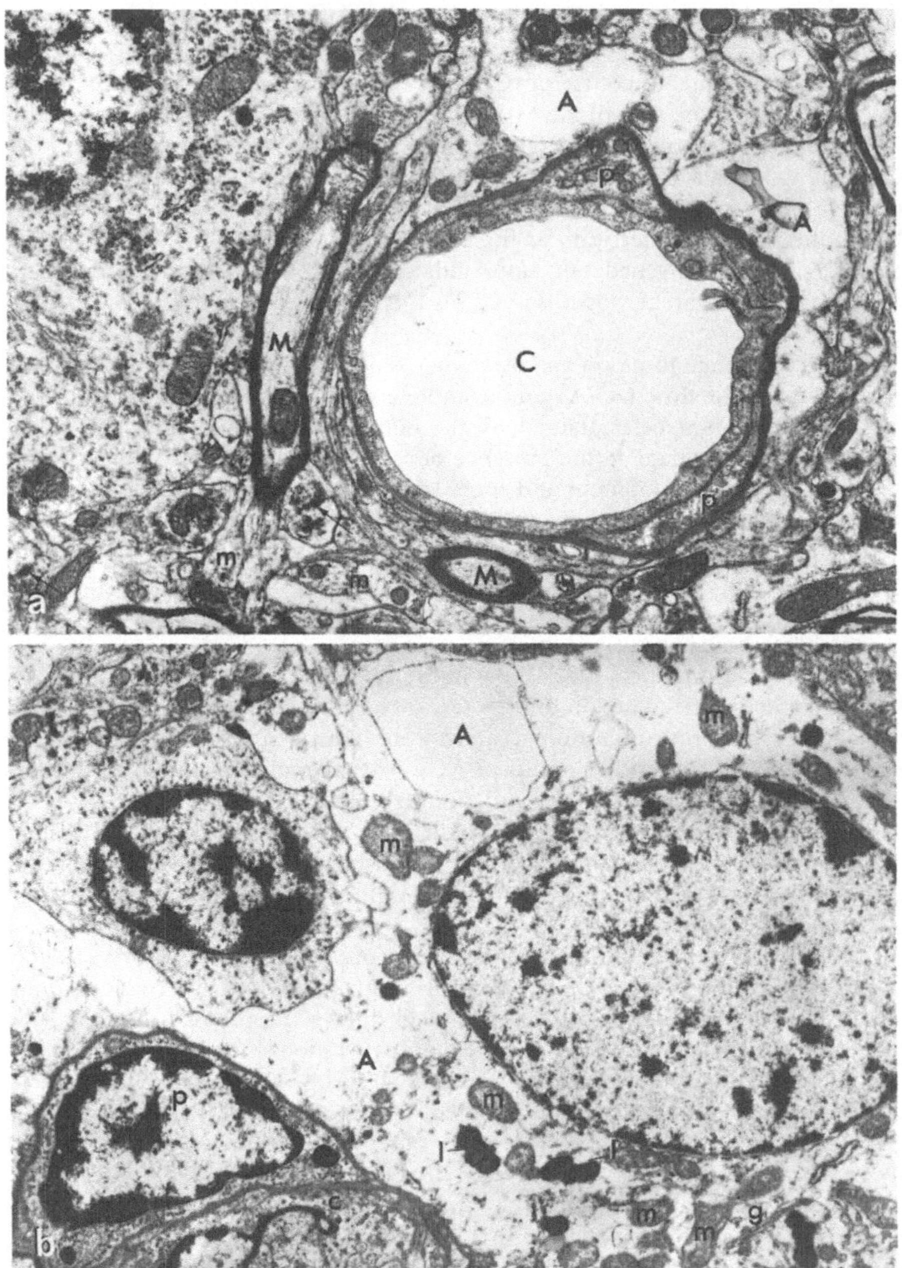

Fig. 11a–c. Electronmicroscopic studies during course of ischemic edema following MCA occlusion in the monkey

a 2 hours after occlusion. Early cytotoxic phase with swollen astrocyte (A) and intact capillary (C) and pericytic (P) structures. Intact myelinated (M) and unmyelinated (m) fibres

b 6 hours after occlusion. Progressive state of ischemic edema with enlarged astrocytes. Golgi structures (g) and lysosomal elements (l)

c 24 hours after occlusion. Vasogenic state of ischemic edema with fragmentation of all structures

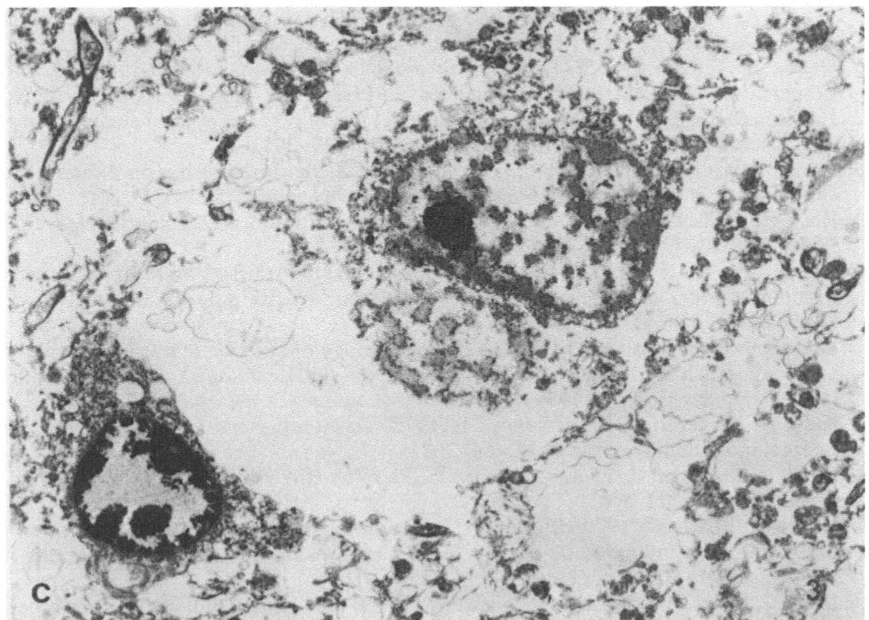

Fig. 11c

that early, continuous administration of high doses of dexamethasone after cerebral infarction might improve restoration of flow and prevent damage to blood flow regulatory mechanisms of the brain. This probably is due to prevention of the spread of edema to tissue which is not directly involved by the ischemic process. Transition of cytotoxic to vasogenic edema type might be influenced also [11, 20]. Figure 11 for instance indicates in three steps the transition from the cytotoxic to the vasogenic type of edema following MCA-occlusion in monkeys. During the early phase of ischemia (Fig. 11a) astrocytes are swollen but the capillaries including the endothelium are intact. During the following hours astrocytes accumulate fluid (Fig. 11b). One day after clip positioning the electronmicroscopic picture indicates the vasogenic type (Fig. 11c) with fragmentation of all structural elements. It might well be that dexamethasone interferes with this morphological course of the ischemic edema.

References

1. Agnoli A, Fieschi C, Bozzao L (1968) Autoregulation of cerebral blood flow. Studies during drug-induced hypertension in normal subjects and in patients with cerebral vascular diseases. Circulation 38:800–812
2. Bartko D, Reulen HJ, Koch H, Schürmann K (1972) Effect of dexamethasone on the early edema following occlusion of the middle cerebral artery in cats. In: Steroids and brain edema. Reulen HJ, Schürmann K (eds). Springer, Berlin Heidelberg New York, pp 127–138
3. De la Torre JC, Surgeon JW (1976) Dexamethasone and DMSO in experimental transorbital cerebral infarction. Stroke 7:577–583
4. Donley RF, Sundt ThM (1973) The effect of dexamethasone on the edema of focal cerebral ischemia. Stroke 4:148–153

5. Fenske A, Fischer M, Regli F, Hase U (1979) The response of focal ischemic cerebral edema to dexamethasone. J Neurol 220:199–209
6. Garcia JH, Lossinsky AS (1979) Cerebrovascular/diseases, introduction 11th Princeton Conference. Price ThR, Nelson E (eds). Raven Press, New York, pp 125–130
7. Harrison MJG, Brownbill D, Lewis PD, Russel RWR (1973) Cerebral edema following carotid artery ligation in the gerbil. Arch Neurol 28:389–391
8. Harrison MJG, Russel RWR (1972) The effect of dexamethasone on experimental cerebral infarction in the gerbil. J Neurol Neurosurg Psychiat 35:520–521
9. Harvey J, Rasmussen T (1951) Occlusion of the middle cerebral artery. Arch Neurol Psychiat 66:20–29
10. Hoppe WE, Waltz AG, Jordan MM, Jacobson RL (1974) Effect of dexamethasone on distribution of water and pertechnetate in brain of cats after middle cerebral artery occlusion. Stroke 5:617–622
11. Hossmann K-A, Schuier FJ (1979) Pathophysiology of stroke edema: In: Brain and heart infarct II. Zülch KJ, Kaufmann W, Hossmann KA, Hossmann V (eds). Springer, Berlin Heidelberg New York, pp 119–129
12. Kahn K, Franarone GF, Newman Th (1972) Dexamethasone treatment of experimental cerebral infarction. Neurology 22:406–407
13. Katzman R, Clasen R, Klatzo I, Meyer JS, Pappius HM, Waltz AG (1977) Brain edema in stroke. Stroke 8:509–540
14. Klatzo L, Spatz M (1979) Studies on experimental ischemia in mongolian gerbils. In: Brain and heart infarct II. Zülch KJ, Kaufmann W, Hossmann KA, Hossmann V (eds). Springer, Berlin Heidelberg New York, pp 130–139
15. Lee MC, Mastri AR, Waltz AG, Loewensohn RB (1974) Ineffectiveness of dexamethasone treatment of experimental cerebral infarction. Stroke 5:216–218
16. Little RJ, Kerr WLF, Sundt TM Jr (1974) Significant of neuronal alterations in developing cortical infarction. Mayo Clin Proc 49:827–836
17. Meyer JS (1958) Circulatory changes following occlusion of the middle cerebral artery and their relation to function. J Neurosurg 15:653–673
18. O'Brien M, Waltz A (1973) Transorbital approach for occluding the middle cerebral artery craniectomy. Stroke 4:201–296
19. O'Brien M, Waltz A, Jordan MM (1974) Ischemic brain edema. Arch Neurol 30:456–460
20. Pappius HM (1979) Evolution of edema in experimental cerebral infarction. In: 11th Princeton conference. Price ThR, Nelson E (eds). Raven Press, New York, pp 131–140
21. Patten BM, Mendell J, Bruun B, Cortin W, Carter S (1972) Doubleblind study of the effects of dexamethasone on acute stroke. Neurol 22:377–383
22. Paulson OB (1970) Regional cerebral blood flow in apoplexy due to occlusion of the middle cerebral artery. Neurol 20:63–77
23. Paulson OB, Lassen NA, Skinhoj E (1970) Regional cerebral blood flow in apoplexa without arterial occlusion. Neurol 21:125–138
24. Pollay M (1975) Formation of cerebrospinal fluid. J Neurosurg 42:665–673
25. Siegel BA, Studer RK, Potchen EJ (1972) Effect of dexamethasone on triethyl tin induced brain edema and the early edema in cerebral ischemia. In: Steroids and brain edema. Reulen JH, Schürmann K (eds). Springer, Berlin Heidelberg New York, pp 113–122
26. Sundt TM, Waltz AG (1966) Experimental cerebral infarction: retroorbital extradural approach for occluding the middle cerebral artery. Mayo Clin Proc 41:159–168
27. Symon L (1963) Effects of vascular occlusion on middle cerebral arterial pressure in dogs and Macacus rhesus. J Physiol (Lond.) 165:62–63
28. Symon L (1970) Regional cerebrovascular response to acute ischaemia in normocapnia and hypercapnia. J Neurol Neurosurg Psychiat 33:756–762
29. Symon L, Branston NM, Strong AJ (1976) Autoregulation in acute focal ischemia. Stroke 7:547–554
30. Symon L, Crockard HA, Dorsch NWC, Branston NM, Juhasz J (1972) Local cerebral blood flow and vascular reactivity in a chronic stable stroke in baboons. Stroke 6:482–492
31. Yamaguchi T, Waltz AG, Okazaki H (1971) Hyperemia and ischemia in experimental cerebral infarction: correlation of histopathology and regional blood flow. Neurol 21:565–578

Is Brain Edema Amenable to Treatment?

M. Brock

In former times a distinction was sought between brain swelling (Hirnschwellung) and brain edema (Hirnödem) (Reichardt, 1904). Nowadays a vasogenic edema is contrasted to a cytotoxic (Klatzo, 1967). At all times, however, clinicians as well as men involved in basic research had one common goal: to find an efficient treatment for this (these?) intriguing condition (conditions?), which apparently may have many different causes, and is (are) considered responsible for the most severe degrees of neurologic disfunction. At a second sight, however, this incrimination appears unjustified since, to the best of our knowledge, there is no evidence at all that edema or swelling *per se*, by the simple increase in tissue fluid volume, has any deleterious effect at all on neural activity. This apparently challenging postulate is substantiated by the fact that all experimental "brain edema models" are also accompanied by an impairment of local blood flow. To the clinician, also, it is sometimes surprising to see marked clinical improvement following corticoid therapy despite no reduction (or even an increase) in the hypodense ("edema") zone around a brain tumor on computerized tomography. The above facts, recently reemphasized by Langfitt (1982) led the editors of this volume to compile data contributed by several authors actively involved in studies on the pathophysiology and therapy of brain edema.

Hossmann (this volume) has studied this problem in cats with implanted brain tumors. Using an immunohistochemical technique for staining serum proteins, he demonstrated that peritumoral edema remains strictly within the white matter and does not penetrate the cortex or cross to the contralateral hemisphere through the corpus callosum. This increase in proteins is paralleled by an increase in tissue water content (from 68% to 82% in 2 weeks), in tissue volume (by more than 70%), and by tissue sodium (to 123 mEq). However, there also is a substancial decrease in local (peritumoral) blood flow (by 40%).

Interestingly, Hossmann finds that reduction of tissue flow due to edema is only an apparent one and no longer detectable when flow values are "referred to dry rather than to wet weight". This finding challenges our initial postulate that edema causes damage only through ischemia and consequent hypoxia. The role of the increase in intercapillary distance due to edema remains open in these studies.

Experimental middle cerebral artery occlusion also leads to a rapid increase in tissue volume through progressive swelling. Tissue sodium content is increased, as is tissue impedance. In this case, however, water is mainly intracellular during the first 4 hours (cytotoxic type of edema). This water increase is due to an increase in tissue osmolality and to a decrease in extracellular sodium. Only after 6 hours does this cytotoxic edema become vasogenic. Hossmann believes this transition from

Treatment of Cerebral Edema
Edited by A. Hartmann and M. Brock

cytotoxic to vasogenic edema to be due to tissue necrosis. It follows that any treatment for cerebrovascular occlusion to be effective has to be initiated without delay, and counteract early cytotoxic edema.

The studies of Marmarou (this volume) stress the importance of tissue pressure gradients as propelling force for the propagation and resoprtion of brain edema by bulk flow, as first postulated by us 10 years ago (Pöll et al., 1972) and summarized at the ICP Symposium in Lund (Brock et al. 1975). Marmarou's study, however, also appears to indicate that formation and resolution of brain edema is not only a "hydrostatic" problem, and that extravasated proteins may be, per se, an important factor, as also suggested by Maier-Hauff et al. (this volume). It appears that (at least some) "free" proteins are not well tolerated by brain tissue or may even serve as mediator substances for brain edema. If this applies not only to extravasated serum proteins, but also to those resulting from tissue necrosis, this might well explain Hossmann's observation that "cytotoxic" edema becomes "vasogenic" when tissue necrosis occurs.

The recent finding (Hossmann, 1982) that dexamethasone prevents the decrease in ATP in the presence of brain edema caused by implanted brain tumors in the cat appears to confirm that energetic mechanisms are also involved in brain edema resolution. As shown by Baethmann et al. (this volume) adrenalectomy without steroid substitution in dogs causes an increase in cortical water content (without changes in white matter!), reduction of CBF (without impairment of regulatory mechanisms) and of glucose uptake. These authors consider the brain to be a "target organ" for steroids. However, their findings that corticoids provide an "attenuation of gross blood brain barrier damage" does not appear to be substantiated by te results of Hossmann (1982) in cats with implanted brain tumors.

Another interesting finding of Marmarou (this volume) is that resorption of edema fluid by the "ventricular route" takes place only as long as there is an egress of fluid from the vascular compartment, providing a pressure head for fluid propagation. This, however, implies that additional mechanisms are involved in resolution of brain edema when its extravasation has ceased. This might be the stage at which protein phagocitosis by glial cells comes into play as suggested by Klatzo (1981). The removal of interstitial proteins by glial cells would be accompanied by a decrease in interstitial colloidosmotic pressure. Water freed by this process can return freely to the vascular compartment.

Nevertheless, as pointed out by O'Brien (this volume), several paramters have to be taken into consideration when discussing this subject, mainly from the clinical point of view. *Duration* and *depth* of ischemia, the two factors considered responsible for the extent of the damage and for outcome, are difficult to estimate and depend on numerous known and unknown factors such as recirculation, collaterals, local perfusion pressure, heterogeneity of blood flow distribution, cellular metabolism, etc. This explains the variability of "brain edema symptoms" (Berndt, this volue) as well as the apparently controversial oppinions on the efficiacy of corticoid therapy. It is beyond the scope of this paper to review this matter in detail. However, attention must be drawn to the fact that while there is no doubt that corticoids markedly and promptly improve symptoms caused by peritumoral edema, their efficiency appears to be less marked in the presence of the traumatic edema that accompanies severe head injury. Both forms of edema, however, can be considered

to be of the vasogenic type. The doubtful or "weak" action of corticoids in cases of severe head injury can not be explained by widespread structural (traumatic) damage of cell membranes due to the direct action of impacting forces, since corticoids also appear to fail in influencing the symptoms attributed to the edema associated with acute cerebrovascular occlusion, where such a traumatic damage does not occur. Where, then, lies the difference? Probably the time factor plays a major role by permitting a larger degree of "metabolic reserves" (compensatory mechanisms) to develop when edema comes slowly. Another (at least partial) explanation for the beneficial effects of corticoids in patients with brain tumor may reside in the reduction of periodic pathological variations of ICP (pressure waves) frequently observed in cases of brain tumor (Kullberg and West, 1965; Cabrini et al., 1967; Yamamura et al., 1982) but less frequent in patients with acute head injury or acute cerebrovascular occlusion. By reducing ICP variations, corticoids make cerebral perfusion pressure more constant, a phenomenon known as *barostabilisation* (Brock et al., 1976) thus improving blood supply to the endangered areas of the brain.
The question chosen as title of the present paper, "Is brain edema amenable to treatment?", can not, then, be answered simply by yes *or* nor, but rather by yes *and* no. Logically, two questions follow: (1st) *when* yes and *when* no?, and (2nd) *why* yes and *why* no? To judge from our present knowlede and methodology, there is still some time to go until the answers to these questions will have become clear.

References

Brock M, Furuse M, Weber R, Hasuo M, Dietz H (1975) Brain Tissue Pressure Gradients, In: Lundberg N, Pouten U, Brock M (eds): Intracranial Pressure II. Springer, Berlin Heidelberg New York pp 215–220

Brock M, Wiegand H, Zillig C, Zywietz C, Mock P, Dietz H (1976) The effect of dexamethasone on intracranial pressure in patients with supratentorial tumors. In: Pappius HM, Feindel W (eds): Dynamics of Brain Edema. Springer, Berlin Heidelberg New York pp 330–336

Cabrini GP, Giovanelli M, Infuso L (1967) Influenza del desametazone sulla pressione liquorale ventricolare in casi di ipertensione endocranica. Minerva neurochir (Torino) *11*:94–102

Hossmann KA (1982) New trend for the evaluation of experimental brain edema. Lecture delivered at the Vth International Symposium on Intracranial Pressure Tokyo

Klatzo I (1967) Presidential adress: Neuropathological aspects of brain edema. J Neuropath Exp Neurol *26*: 1–14

Klatzo I (1981) Interrelationships between cerebral blood flow (CBF) and brain edema (BE). Minderhoud JM In: (ed). Cerebral Blood Flow. Basic knowledge and clinical implications. Excerpta Medica, Amsterdam Oxford Princeton pp 160–173

Kullberg G, West KA (1965) Influence of corticosteroids on ventricular fluid pressure. Acta neurol Scand 41 (suppl 13): 445–452

Langfitt T (1982) Comment during the Vth International Symposium on Intracranial Pressure. Tokyo

Pöll W, Brock M, Markakis E, Winkelmüller W, Dietz H (1972) Brain Tissue Pressure. In: Brock M, Dietz H (eds): Intracranial Pressure. Springer, Berlin Heidelberg New York pp 188–194

Reichardt M (1905) Zur Entstehung des Hirndrucks bei Hirngeschwülsten und anderen Hirnkrankheiten und über eine bei diesen zu beobachtende besondere Art der Hirnschwellung. Dtsch Z Nervenheilk *28*: 306–355
Yamamura A, Saeki N, Nakamura T, Isobe K, Watanabe Y, Makino H (1982) Distribution of pressure waves A&B in 24-hours-period of day in patients with brain tumor and effects of steroid. Contribution to the Vth International Symposium on Intracranial Pressure. Tokyo

Subject Index

Advances in Neurosurgery

Volume 10

Computerized Tomography – Brain Metabolism – Spinal Injuries

Editors: W. Driesen, M. Brock, M. Klinger
1982. 186 figures, 76 tables. Approx. 420 pages
ISBN 3-540-11115-8

Contents: Computerized Tomography. – Brain Metabolism. – Spinal Injuries. – Free Topics. – Subject Index.

Volume 9

Brain Abscess and Meningitis Subarachnoid Hemorrhage: Timing Problems

Editors: W. Schiefer, M. Klinger, M. Brock
1981. 219 figures, 134 tables. XIX, 519 pages
ISBN 3-540-10539-5

Contents: Brain Abscess and Meningitis. – Subarachnoid Hemorrhage: Timing Problems. – Free Topics. – Subject Index.

Volume 8

Surgery of Cervical Myelopathy Infantile Hydrocephalus: Long-Term Results

Editors: W. Grote, M. Brock, H.-E. Clar, M. Klinger, H. E. Nau
1980. 178 figures in 215 separate illustrations, 138 tables. XVII, 456 pages
ISBN 3-540-09949-2

Contents: Cervical Myelopathy. – Hydrocephalus in Childhood. – Free Topics. – Subject Index.

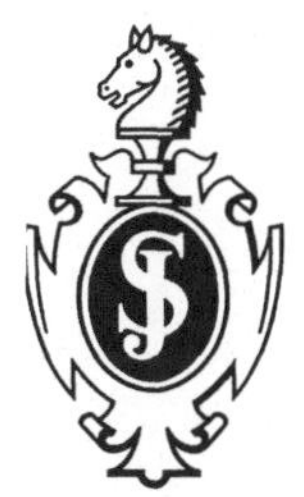

Springer-Verlag
Berlin
Heidelberg
New York

Modern Neurosurgery 1

Editor: M. Brock
1982. 158 figures, 95 tables. XIV, 484 pages
ISBN 3-540-10972-2

Contents: Technical Developments. – Head Injury-Intensive Care. – Chemotherapy of Brain Tumours. – Surgery of the Pituitary Region. – Surgery of Ventricular Tumours. – Spinal Cord. – Reconstructive Vascular Surgery. – Vasospasm. – Aneurysm Surgery. – Functional Neurosurgery. – Subject Index.

MODERN NEUROSURGERY is a new Springer-Verlag series whose volumes appear at four-year intervals. The editor of Modern Neurosurgery is the Editor of Congress Publications of the World Federation of Neurosurgical Societies (WFNS). Each volume contains about 50 papers selected from the several hundred submitted to the corresponding WFNS Congress.
The aim of MODERN NEUROSURGERY is to provide a precise and broad overview of the state of art of Neurosurgery as viewed by international authorities.

Microsurgery for Cerebral Ischemia

Editors: S. J. Peerless, C. W. McCormick
1980. 282 figures. XVII, 372 pages
ISBN 3-540-90495-6

Treatment of Hydrocephalus Computer Tomography

Editors: R. Wüllenweber, H. Wenker, M. Brock, M. Klinger
1978. 111 figures, 86 tables. XXXI, 230 pages
(Advances in Neurosurgery, Volume 6)
ISBN 3-540-09031-2

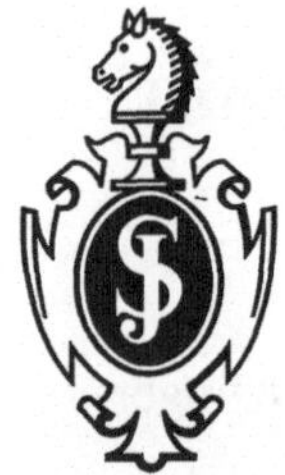

Springer-Verlag
Berlin
Heidelberg
New York

Dynamics of Brain Edema

Proceedings of the 3rd International Workshop on Dynamic Aspects of Cerebral Edema, Montreal, Canada, June 25–29, 1976
Editors: H. M. Pappius, W. Feindel
1976. 83 figures, 81 tables. XIII, 404 pages
ISBN 3-540-08009-0